I0440388

It's Your Body - You're the One In It

Take Control of Your Own Health and Healing

Carl Brahe MA

Copyright © 2014 Carl Brahe

All rights reserved.

ISBN-13: 978-1499158304

DEDICATION

Dedicated to my wife Victoria who helps me discover my missing pieces and heal my wounded parts.

CONTENTS

Acknowledgments   vi

INTRODUCTION   vii

Chapter 1   **IT'S MY BODY AND I'M THE ONE IN IT**   1

Sleep Apnea   3

Life Challenges   6

Taking Responsibility No Matter What   8

Want/Don't Want   8

Chapter 2   **SOFT BODY APPROACH TO MIND/BODY HEALING**   11

Life Energy   13

The Soft Body   15

Your Soft Body   16

Vibrant Truth   18

The Silent Witness   19

Awareness and Intent   20

Grounding   23

Grounding II   25

Grounding to the Opposite   25

Mindfulness   26

Wu Wei   26

Where Is the Center of Your Universe?   27

We All Share the Same Water   27

The Eagle   28

Boundaries   29

Perceiving Body Energy   30

The Power of Touch   31

When Does a Touch Begin?   32

Unruffling   33

Healing Water   34

Expansion and Contraction Exercise   35

Chapter 3   **REALMS OF HEALING**   37

Relationship   37

The Inner Child   44

Spiritual   45

Dreams   49

The Birth Council   51

I Am   52

Protecting Yourself 53

Loss of Self 54

Reclaiming Your Energy 55

Community Mind 57

Emotional 58

Beliefs and Emotions 59

Anatomy of Anger 61

Boundaries of Belief; The Prison of Emotion 62

Intellectual 66

The Secret 67

Self-Talk 67

Affirmations 68

Belief 72

Verbal Probes 74

Draw Your Beliefs 75

Physical 76

Working with the Physical Body 77

Squeaky Wheel 78

Yoga Nidra 79

Personifying the Pain 81

PTSD and Moral Injury   83

Love Yourself if You Can   84

Precious Pain   84

Dance with Pain   88

Healing Without Content   88

Inspection Tour   89

Chapter 4   **EXERCISE WITH NO PAIN,**   93
               CONSTANT GAIN

I Love Recess   93

Dancing with Weights   98

Aspirin   100

Breath   101

Breathing Exercises   101

Sound   103

Toning   104

Chapter 5   **TECHNIQUES**   107

Sensitivity Cycle   107

Relaxation   109

Imagery   110

A Safe Place   111

Light   116

Bone Marrow Cleansing   118

Organ Cleansing and Charging   119

Core of Energy   119

Make it Fun   120

Participating in Your Medical Treatment   120

ABOUT THE AUTHOR   125

ACKNOWLEDGMENTS

Thanks to the amazing faculty and students of Boulder Graduate School. Thanks to Debbie Bernhard for bringing my focus back to this work.

INTRODUCTION

Dealing with illness or injury can be very confusing. There are so many opinions available on the web, from friends, family and healthcare professionals. Traditional medical practitioners may disagree with alternative practitioners, who are likely to disagree with each other. All these people may have something useful to offer or they may all be wrong.

Regardless of whose advice you take, or whose opinion you accept, you are the one responsible, the one who will suffer the consequences of being wrong. You are the one who experiences your body and mind first-hand. Your body can provide reliable guidance to healing and growth if you learn to listen with your inner ear, see with your mind's eye and feel the knowing in your gut.

We have incredible capacities to heal from a wide range of health challenges. Our ability to heal is so incredible that it's amazing when we don't heal. Our bodies must die at some point to maintain the natural flow of birth and death, but until the final shutdown our bodies are normally able to heal almost anything.

Healing is what we naturally do. It's hard wired, but some people heal faster and more completely than others. Two normally healthy people with the same cold may have very different experiences. One may end up in deep misery, staying in bed for several days. The other may hardly notice she has a cold and her life is not at all disrupted. At other times they may experience the opposite. This eBook presents information, meditations, visualizations and exercises to help you heal more quickly and completely from all your life challenges. The emphasis is on helping you discover within yourself the controls that you have to influence your healing both positively and negatively.

You have firsthand experience of your physical and mental states. You have sensory awareness to check inside to see if a diagnosis feels true to your experience. I was a passenger in a car that was broadsided and smashed to half its width. I had two ribs that were totally broken. I could feel the jagged edges brushing past each other when I walked. In the emergency room, after a couple hour wait, I was told that I had no broken ribs. The doctor had consulted with a radiologist to be sure. When I looked at the x-ray I saw two clean breaks in the ribs I had told the doctor were broken. I asked about these two ribs and he seemed amazed to find them broken. He said that my symptoms indicated that the two ribs directly below the broken ones were broken. He, and the radiologist, missed the two that were clearly broken. I believe that the training received by the doctor, and the radiologist, kept them from seeing the reality even when it was pointed out. Even though advances in knowledge are happening so quickly, Michael Gershon, medical professor at Stanford University who discovered that our brains are actually more concentrated in our guts than our skulls, tells his new students that half of what he teaches them will be proven wrong over the next 5 years. Medical professionals have a huge investment in what they have been taught. It's hard for any of us to see that which contradicts our beliefs. We all have a bias to believe our beliefs rather than our experiences and we tend to hold onto beliefs tenaciously even when evidence indicates we are mistaken.

Your mind/body has capacities to experience and influence your life in ways you will probably never comprehend or even discover. You may never understand how your body and mind work but you can learn to direct them to create the outcomes you want. Your mind/body follows your intent. You can learn to be aware of your body's indicators and to consciously influence your own healing process. This eBook will help you to consciously guide your own physical, psychological and spiritual healing processes. It's your body and you're the one in it.

Our immune systems are greater than any model yet suggested, though in the past Western medicine embraced the human immune system with a very limited view. Doctors emphasized the chemical actions of the immune system almost to the exclusion of other medical approaches. They manipulated the electrochemical dynamics (medicines) as the most common treatment of immune related problems. In extreme cases body parts were removed, restructured or destroyed by surgery, chemotherapy or radiation therapy.

Medical professionals are now investigating subtle, and noninvasive, means to boost the human immune system. Different methods of healing that have been explored throughout history are now being rediscovered. French physician, A. A. Tomatis, used the chanting of Gregorian monks to prove that sound stimulates and strengthens the immune system. Dr. Tomatis suggests that immune systems improve when they are fed and charged with nourishing sound.

Osteopaths, nurses, massage therapists and chiropractors use touch and movement to stimulate neural, blood and endocrine flows. The works of Dolores Krieger, Ph.D., Brugh Joy, M.D., and Barbara

Brennan, M.S., show the immune system is affected by what Brennan calls the human energy field. Robert O. Becker, M.D., has measured this energy field in his research. These and other energy healers suggest the intent of the healing practitioner, patient, family and friends directly affects the energetic aspects of immune function. Ancient energy healing practices such as qigong and acupuncture support this view.

The works of O. Carl Simonton, M.D., and Bernie Siegel, M.D., show that belief, emotion and intent directly affect the immune system. They found that you can explore and alter your intent toward healing by using your imagination. Candace Pert, Ph.D., and her associates demonstrated the role of peptides in communicating emotion, belief, and intent at a cellular level.

The use of light in healing also is an ancient practice. In recent times, major research by Russian scientists involved the use of bioplasma (living energy or life energy) and biophotons (light emitted from each body cell) to accelerate healing and cellular regeneration.

These, and aspects yet to be discovered, directly affect your immune system. In this eBook we will explore and experience ways to boost your immune system which are not commonly used in western medicine. The exercises in this book are not intended to replace any medical treatment. Physicians are highly trained professionals. They have an understanding of the specific dynamics of physiology and treatments that are beyond those of us without such training. This work supports and supplements both traditional medicine and alternative treatments.

Use this material along with the vast professional resources available to increase your options when facing major, or minor, life challenges. Use your first-hand experience to foster greater cooperation with your physicians and other healing professionals. The cooperative climate among those in the healing arts is changing. For example, a modern pain center today may include a neurologist, internist, anesthesiologist, surgeon, psychiatrist, psychotherapist, hypnotherapist, spiritual therapist, osteopath, nurse, chiropractor, yoga instructor, biofeedback and relaxation therapist, massage and movement therapist, art therapist, music therapist, physical therapist, social worker and nutritionist. Use all that you need. Allow your inner guidance to find what's right for you.

Perhaps your life challenges are the real source of your ability to live and become stronger. Psychiatrist Milton Erickson often told his patients that he didn't want them to heal too soon, before they reaped the benefits of their life challenges. He taught them that within the problem is an accurate guide to the solution. And, if the person approached the problem as a friend, instead of an enemy, he might find the resources to solve the problem permanently.

It's easy to see how your relationship with the stresses in your world affects healing and growth. Your relationship with stress affects your body like stress affects your car. If you drive your car with anger, you drastically increase energy use in the form of fuel consumed to get to your destination. Driving while angry causes more wear and tear and increases the odds of being in an accident. Prolonged anger does damage to your body and makes you more accident prone. If you go through life fueled by anger, fear, guilt, hatred, etc., you drain your life energy and cause excess wear on your body. These emotions are common and powerful motivating forces in our society. Unfortunately, these also are common attitudes toward healing. You have an inner guidance. This inner guidance may take any form and can provide the creative energy to aid in self-healing. The act of seeking guidance carries an innate intent to discover your resources for healing and how to best use them. It isn't important to know how this works.

A life fueled by loving respect fosters health and healing. As you travel through this eBook, choose to fuel your journey with self-respect and compassion for yourself. The intent of this eBook is self-empowerment, self-respect and self-responsibility. All have a direct effect on your immune system.

Carl Brahe

There is no such thing as a problem without a gift for you in its hands.

Richard Bach, Illusions

PREFACE

Where is your awareness right now? Part of your awareness is present with reading, and processing, these words. You also may be aware of other thoughts and sensations. What percentage is aware of the past or future? What percentage is here in the moment?

A part of your awareness may be thinking about something that happened earlier today, yesterday or in the distant past. Another part might be daydreaming of the future. In our fast-paced lives, we often find it difficult to be present for even a moment. We use a variety of strategies to find safety in a sometimes impossible world. One common strategy involves creating an illusion of not existing in the here, and now, where it might be dangerous to our egos, emotions or bodies. On a certain level of our consciousness, we believe that if we distract ourselves from being present in the moment, we become invisible and therefore safe. By investing our awareness in our thoughts and daydreams, we create and maintain the illusion of safety in the moment.

In a story about the Buddha, he was asked what made him the Buddha, "Are you an angel?" They asked. "No," replied the Buddha. "Are you a god then?" They asked. "No," he replied, "I am simply awake." Being awake is another way of saying being present. In Ayurveda, the system of medicine native to India, the practitioners believe true healing is awakening to the essence of your true self which is a divine (universal) being and is discovered by presence.

If a person who reads this eBook becomes more present and aware of her life energy, this work has succeeded in its mission. The emphasis is on guiding you to experience this essence firsthand. You will learn how to use your life energy to heal and create in the world. I want to stress that I am not implying anyone can heal every disease and ailment. Mystics, gurus, medicine men, medicine women and other healers get the same diseases as everyone else. They grow old and die, like everyone else.

You have the natural ability to heal. You can consciously direct, and participate in, your own healing when you are in the present with any life challenge, when you dispense with the limitations of judgment or disbelief, when you have the clear intent to heal. You can use this presence to aid in your healing whether you are using traditional or alternative medicine. Our flow of consciousness affects our physical bodies like the flow of a river is directed by placing rocks in the river bed. The rocks are our thoughts. They represent our true intent. Brain researchers estimate a person thinks around 60,000 thoughts a day. This is like putting 60,000 rocks a day into the river of our lives to make it flow in the way we choose. Ninety-five percent of these thoughts are the same as we had yesterday. We use a lot of energy day after day picking up these rocks and returning them to the same place.

Thoughts are like the directors in the creation of the molecules of your body. Think back to a few years ago. The body you have now is similar to the one you had then. Your body replaces many of its cells every year; you get an entirely new body every few years. The body you had a few years ago no longer exists. Although most of your body is constantly being replaced, you probably make few changes. Your body recreates itself directed by mostly the same thoughts, beliefs, attitudes and emotions repeated over and over again. Candace Pert's research found that all the instructions at a cellular level to grow, or die, or reproduce, or do anything, are delivered in the form of emotion. Moods and emotions have a direct effect on your body. Witness when you feel blue, or down, how it affects your stance, posture and movement. Someone who has been beaten down by life has a body that reflects his dismal outlook.

Being in the present, with a clear intent to heal, helps clear the rocks in your stream of consciousness which contribute to the creation and maintenance of disease and emotional problems. These problems will be referred to in this eBook as life challenges. The following chapters will help you discover and therefore change some of the beliefs, emotions and energy dynamics that feed and maintain your life challenge. You will discover your inner guidance and learn how to follow it.

Our thoughts reflect our true intent in life. These thoughts flavor the expression of the DNA molecules as we create new cells. Newly emerging body cells are similar until they adopt the role of a specific type of cell. At the time they choose a job, so to speak, they may take on any of the billions of different functions from brain tissue to fingernails. Our thoughts, emotions and intentions affect our health and healing at a cellular level. You can learn to use your thoughts to improve the quality of your life, health and healing.

CHAPTER 1
IT'S MY BODY AND I'M THE ONE IN IT

Many years ago on a summer evening, I pulled up to a four-way stop on a country highway. I paused on my motorcycle and took time to notice the beauty of the surrounding countryside. As I started toward the intersection to make a left turn, I caught a glimpse of another motorcycle in my mirror, tires screaming and brakes locked, coming right at me. An instant later its handlebars slammed into my lower back, the motorcycle flipped over my left hip and tumbled end over end through the intersection and into the ditch.

The next day, I felt extreme pain in my lower back. I knew I needed help. I grew up in a family where we went to see doctors only when we needed vaccinations or had serious injuries. As a result, I didn't trust doctors. After ten days, my wife finally persuaded me to see a chiropractor. I trusted chiropractors even less than medical doctors. Still, I reasoned that they deal with the spine and I needed help, the pain was getting too much to bear.

I found an exceptional chiropractor, named Bent. He had me fill out many forms. One form had a long checklist of about one hundred and fifty symptoms. I checked most of them. Bent looked at me as if to say, I've got another hypochondriac to deal with here. However, after taking a series of X-rays, he said that he was amazed I could walk into his office, and he told me the grim news. He didn't see how I could walk even before the accident. The X-rays showed fused vertebrae. We came to the conclusion that my vertebrae had probably fused because of an automobile accident I was in at age five. Now, because of the recent motorcycle injury, Bent said that if I received a hard slap on my back, or a slight rear end car collision, I would likely become paralyzed. He said, "If your body was a house, I wouldn't step inside. A strong gust of wind might collapse it."

I asked him how I should go about healing the wounds. Bent said it was impossible. He tried, tactfully, to tell me that within ten years life in a wheelchair was almost a certainty.

I asked, "If it was possible, how could I go about repairing the damage?"

To appease me, he showed me the X-rays again. He pointed to the most serious injury that threatened to sever my spinal cord. He reminded me of his findings which showed two vertebrae fused from the childhood injury. These two fused vertebrae are where I chose to start. That was the only part of what Bent told me that I understood.

I asked, "How can I clean these vertebrae of calcium allowing them to move again?"

"Surgery is the only way." he insisted.

I told him, "I'm only interested in how a human body might do it if a human body could." He answered with the guess that somehow the calcium would be carried off and eliminated one grain at a time. The same way it was deposited there.

I began to picture tiny beings inside my body whose job was to handle the transfer of calcium to be used or discarded. I called these beings terriers and talked to them every day. I told them they had been lazy, or forgetful, and had been leaving this calcium lying around where it hindered my back.

In my mind, I continually heard the song, *Working in the Coal Mine*. In every spare moment, I imagined the terriers working to the song, diligently removing the calcium. I checked in (scanned my spine with my awareness) several times a day to keep track of their progress. With my mind's eye, I saw the mass of calcium growing smaller. This translated to the real world with the fact that my vertebrae were slowly beginning to move again. After eighteen months the calcium had dissolved to a thumbnail-shaped sliver and I felt a piercing pain when I moved my back. It felt like an upper vertebrae was grinding against the sharp calcium ridge on the lower vertebrae.

I accepted the pain as a sign of definite progress. Although, after a couple months of being in constant companionship with the pain, I had myself convinced that it could be a tumor. I returned to my chiropractor for new X-rays. Bent was on vacation and at my insistence his replacement took X-rays. After retaking the X-rays several times, he gave me the bad news. He showed me the sliver of calcium digging into my vertebrae and suggested I find a neurosurgeon, fast. I was delighted. He couldn't understand my joy. The X-rays confirmed what my inner senses told me. I was healing. My terriers were sent back to work with renewed vigor. After a couple of months, the pain gradually disappeared.

About a year-and-a-half after the accident I jokingly asked Bent, "Is it okay for me to go skydiving now?"

"Only idiots jump out of airplanes!" He snapped. He told me that sky-diving presents a danger for permanent back and ankle injury for anyone. He finished with telling me, "There is no medical reason that you shouldn't skydive, if that's what you want to do."

I was shocked." I thought you told me I'd wind up in a wheelchair right after my first landing." I said.

He said that he would never have believed it possible, but I had healed well enough in his opinion that he felt I could do anything I chose. What impressed me was that my back had healed in spite of the chiropractor's diagnosis, even though his prediction wasn't something that I ever believed. What amazed me most, my thirty-year old injuries also had healed!

I was able to heal as a result of the combination of Bent's healing skills and my willingness to do the required work daily. My healing surprised him. He couldn't understand why I had healed from this type of injury. Through hindsight, I realize that the calcium that fused the vertebrae together acted as a natural cast which allowed my childhood injury to heal.

Over the years I have used these techniques for many reasons and they have seldom failed me. I've found it effective for accelerating healing of all kinds. Sleep apnea is one challenge I found these techniques to be very effective for me for treating without drugs, machines or surgery.

Sleep Apnea

When I was 49-years-old I was diagnosed with sleep apnea that was so severe that I was told I might die any moment from heart attack or stroke. When I was sleeping, I only breathed for 20 minute out of an hour. My pulse and blood oxygen levels dropped dangerously low every night. The more I slept the more tired I became. To me it felt like every time I went to sleep someone suffocated me almost to the point of death but gave me just enough oxygen to stay alive. At one point I was so tired, and my body ached so much, and my brain was so foggy, that if someone had offered to shoot me in the head I would have said, "Yes, please."

I don't know how long the apnea had been happening. It was

diagnosed more than a decade after I found myself at an intersection in a neighborhood I knew well wondering where I was and how I got there. The most common cause of death for those with apnea is falling asleep while driving. At that time I fell asleep every time I sat down. For years, I was passed around from doctor to doctor, each with a theory, but none were right. In the time it took to diagnose the apnea my hands and forearms, feet and ankles, went numb. Every muscle in my body constantly burned from oxygen deprivation. Thinking was painful. My organs were shutting down as my body withdrew oxygen from non-essential areas to maintain heart function. I was literally dying, being slowly suffocated.

I was handed off to a head surgeon who thought I might have a hairline crack in my skull from unknown origin. As an afterthought he said, "This is probably a long shot but I'm going to send you to the sleep lab." It took them less than 5 minute to diagnose apnea and within a couple days it was confirmed by a sleep study.

I was prescribed a bi-pap machine which made things worse. I couldn't sleep at all with it. I told the doctor that I couldn't use it and he said I had to. I told him I wouldn't use it. He said I had to because it was doctors' orders and the medical supply company would not even take the machine back without his order. I told him I was going to do it my way. He finally said with a smirk, okay we'll give you a month and do another sleep study. He warned me that apnea was incurable and only treatable with bi-pap machines and/or surgery. The follow-up sleep study, a month later, showed only borderline apnea with no need for treatment. No one in the sleep clinic asked what I had done. It didn't fit into their beliefs.

I did some research to learn about apnea. My understanding was that when I slept my soft palate would collapse and block my throat so air couldn't flow until it became a life and death struggle that resulted in waking with a loud gasp.

I decided that there were three main areas that I needed to work on:

1. I had to strengthen my soft palate. I discovered from trial and error that toning made my soft palate stretch and form different shapes using vowel sounds. Chanting, or a more forceful sounding, increased the intensity of the palate

movement. Movement equaled strengthening in my mind.

2. I needed to strengthen my diaphragm and learn to breath deeper to increase breath pressure making it harder to shut off my throat with a weak palate. I started with deep breathing, visualizing my breath dropping so low into my body that the bottoms of my feet expanded when I inhaled. Another exercise I used was breathing deep into my pelvis, then expel the breath with the image of rolling up my diaphragm like a toothpaste tube. Also, very useful was singing, or chanting, while exercising my abdomen. Riding a bicycle uphill, using a stair master or an ellipse machine while singing is an example. Any strenuous exercise will work. The act of controlling your breath to maintain a steady air flow required to sing builds diaphragm strength, as well as, strengthening core muscles.

3. I had to find a way to be aware when I quit breathing while sleeping. I used mindfulness mediation with the wordless intent to learn this awareness along with intending before I went to sleep to wake if I was not breathing or if I was snoring.

One of the basics of mind/body healing is that every physical malady has an emotional aspect that is inseparable from the physical. Expressing the emotional aspect is one way to release it. One way to do this is to sound out the emotion. Make whatever sound it feels like. If it feels like a scream, scream. If it feels like a song, sing it. Whatever you find, express it. Anger and fear are common. Expressing these things may sound and feel rageful or terrifying. Let them out with no judgment. Let it be an interesting phenomenon.

Using these techniques I have been free of apnea for over 10 years. Rehabbing my body and brain function has been a slower process. Rebuilding muscles and rejuvenating organs for me has been a painful process that involved challenging my mind and body daily one inch and one pebble at a time. I made it fun so I would stick with it. The physical exercise section has more on that. For several years, I had the sensation of surfacing after a deep dive under water, with oxygen running out, and vision coming in dark waves, the surface always coming closer but never reaching it. My brain, and the rest of my body, seemed to be screaming for air. After many months, I felt like I surfaced one day, and my body finally had enough air. My brain function began to improve, and my endurance, and muscles, grew as the constant pain subsided.

Everyone has unique life challenges, and our healing process are different, but if you take charge of your own healing, you will heal more quickly and completely than if you don't. By taking charge of your own healing, using your own sensory experiences to guide you, along with appropriate professional help, you will create a better healing outcome. Your medical team usually only sees you for a few minutes at a time and make the best judgments they know how to. If you allow your health to be dependent on others doing the healing work for you ("My doctors don't seem to be able to get it right.") you are giving control to those who don't have the stake in success that you do. It's your body and your health.

Life Challenges

What exactly is a life challenge? Throughout your life there are barriers. There are barriers to having what you want and being happy. Barriers sometimes exist against having satisfying and nurturing relationships. During your life you will encounter barriers that limit your quality of life in some way. I call these barriers life challenges.

Most life challenges result from beliefs and emotional charges that we attach to different areas of our lives. Some challenges may be physical, such as cancer or multiple sclerosis, but most are less concrete, less life threatening. Some life challenges are emotional charges: anger, hate, jealousy, greed and so on. Even subtle life challenges, related to forgotten hurts, and fears, can create problems in our everyday lives.

It's not hard to see how our relationships with life affect our health. If you live stressfully most of the time, your constant overreaction may lead to stroke, ulcers, cancer or heart attack. If you are depressed, so is your immune system and brain function. If you lack self-respect, it will probably be reflected in the food, and other substances, you consume. The way you feel about yourself affects the way you treat yourself.

In short, a life challenge is anything that interferes with living in a deeply satisfying and fulfilling way.

My back injury provided the opportunity to heal the earlier

emotional and physical life challenge associated with my fused vertebrae. Surgery became unnecessary; my body removed the fused calcium. As my spine healed, I worked through some childhood traumas, and released many old beliefs, emotions, and attitudes. My lifestyle changed, so did the way I treated myself and others. The quality of my relationships was changing as well. Ignoring my doctor's beliefs, I chose to heal myself. I used the tools that were natural and easily available to me - music, imagery and the willingness to change.

The changes touched every area of my life. They happened without my being aware of their scope. Now I work with what my mind, body and spirit present to me. I follow the guidance that occurs naturally by the process of working toward an active and healthier life. The changes that grew out of this movement toward healing created a robust, stronger me. The changes continue 30 years later.

A series of exercises to become aware of your natural inner guidance are included in this eBook. These exercises will help you learn to use your firsthand experience to discover and use your inner resources. The purpose of the exercises is to acquaint you with how your health is affected by your relationships with your inner and outer worlds. Each exercise is designed so you can see and learn ways to control your immune function. Like riding a bicycle, the real learning is in the experience. You can talk about it until you understand every detail of how to do it. Yet, until you get on the bike, fall and get up several times, you really won't know and feel the experience of controlling the bicycle. With these exercises, you won't skin your knee. They are only meant to increase your awareness of your natural resources. You experience what you experience, and that is all that's important. You may do these exercises anytime or anyplace. Use parts of the exercises or expand them to fit your needs.

Approach these exercises with ease and a sense of humor. They are many times more effective if you have fun with them. Don't force anything. Being tense and desperate are obstacles to your healing process. The only strife in healing is what we project on it with our beliefs and emotions. Learning to relax, laugh and let go are your friends.

Taking Responsibility No Matter What

A toddler had been severely injured by her mother who smashed her daughter's skull leaving the child severely disabled. A nurse who cared for the child asked me who was responsible. I told her the child was. She asked how that could possibly be. I told her that practically speaking, if the child accepted responsibility, it allowed her to focus all her energy on healing, instead of being hindered by fear and blame. The child did nothing to deserve what happened to her, but if she didn't accept responsibility she would always be a victim, and healing would be much more challenging, if not impossible. Her healing energy would be wasted on victimhood.

In our lives we face many challenges. If we choose to take responsible, no matter what happens, we are in a position to do something about it. If we are victims, we have little, or no, power to change our situation. When we approach a life challenge as a powerless victim, we automatically surrender to it, investing our life energy in nourishing and perpetuating it. Many life challenges require a long term commitment to work diligently, without blame, for a long period of time, to bring about a healthy resolution. This may require a great deal of energy and concentration. Blaming, whining and revenge are just a waste of your precious energy. If you get knocked down, regardless of how or why, you have two choices. You can lie there and talk to yourself about how bad things, are or you can get up, and continue living your life.

Want/Don't Want

If you ask the average person what she/he wants, the reply will almost always be in the form of don't want. If you ask, "What do you want out of life?" The reply will most likely start with, "Well, I don't want this." If you press for what the person does want, it will probably lead to increasing frustration, possibly with an insistence that, "What I want is what I don't want." The person will probably not use these words, but the message is, "I know what I don't want and that defines what I do want."

Don't want defines only what you don't want, and focusing your energy on don't want will bring what you don't want. If you spend your life avoiding what you don't want, getting what you do want will happen only by accident. Moving away from what you don't want, will probably not result in moving toward what you do want.

When you change your focus to what you want in life, you direct your energy toward accomplishing what you do want. Focusing on what you want makes you aware of the opportunities to create what you want in your life. If you focus on what you don't want, you will find opportunities to create what you don't want.

Chapter 2

SOFT BODY APPROACH TO MIND/BODY HEALING

Psychoneuroimmunology (PNI) is the study, and practice, of actively, and consciously, participating in, and directing, our own healing. Psycho refers to the mind, or our ability to choose, or to have intent. Neuro refers to the brain and nervous system. Immunology refers to the body's natural immune defenses such as white blood cells, T-cells and macrophages. PNI also is the study of how, and why, we directly influence our healing with our beliefs and emotions. This is another name for mind/body healing.

The practice of PNI is not new. Many ancient cultures and religions used similar healing techniques. The Taoist priests of China collected more than sixteen hundred volumes on an energy transformative form of healing called Qigong.

The modern study of PNI started, in this country, in the late 1950's. An amazing boy in a hospital in Massachusetts shocked the western world's medical community. He had an inoperable, grapefruit-sized brain tumor that was growing larger every day. His family felt each trip to the hospital might be his last.

The boy intuitively began to play a game in his mind. He imagined white space ships flying around in his brain, blasting his tumor with beams of light. In the following weeks he not only imagined the tumor away, but baffled the medical world by his remarkable recovery. As the tumor shrunk in his imagination, so did the tumor in his brain.

During the early stages of research, the practice of PNI was crude. Most psychoneuroimmunology (PNI) practice involved imagining white blood cells in some symbolic form. They imagined space ships, white knights or white dogs attacking and killing the invading forces of the disease. At first, the little boy's space ship format was followed by others since it was the only well-documented case of spontaneous remission available to investigators. Researchers soon added hypnosis, guided imagery and meditation to PNI. The heightened sensitivity caused by these altered states of awareness began to shed light on the emotional and energetic aspects of the human immune system.

Researchers discovered that the white blood cells, and all other

11

body cells, have receptor sites for the same neurotransmitters that signal emotion in the brain. Candace Pert's neuropeptide studies suggest that the cells in your immune system feel the same emotions as you feel. If you are depressed, every aspect of your being, including your immune system, becomes depressed. The opposite is also true.

In absence of other medical options, using belief in the form of a placebo to aid healing is an honored tradition in the medical community. A placebo is a kind of trick used by doctors. The medication has no known medical effects, yet, in a surprising number of cases the person recovers even when they know they are taking a placebo. Placebos have provided remarkable healings since the beginning of recorded history. Most doctors use them successfully throughout their careers.

Today, PNI involves the study of systemic disease by way of two opposing medical approaches. The allopathic, or traditional, approach is mainly concerned with your body's electrochemical properties. Doctors change specific balances with drugs and medical technology to help restore you to health. For instance, antibiotics fight bacterial infections by wiping out most of the infectious bacteria. Killing the harmful bacteria gives the helpful bacteria a chance to reestablish itself. This is like poisoning a lake to kill the sucker fish so the trout can survive. It's like shaking one side of a mobile to untangle the strings on the opposite side.

The homeopathic approach helps restore you to health by strengthening weak body systems by stimulating them directly. If you go to a homeopath with a bacterial infection, he might give you something to increase the helpful bacteria. The good bacteria subdues the infectious bacteria and brings the person back to a healthful condition.

This is similar to adding weight to an undersized figure on a mobile in order to create balance. If your liver function is poor, a doctor of homeopathy might give you a potion that supplies the frequency of energetic vibration which is needed to bring the liver back to health. It's as if the vibration of the potion resonates with something in the liver and causes an energetic reaction. When you strike a tuning fork and bring it close to another tuning fork of the same frequency, the unstruck tuning fork starts to vibrate and produce sound.

One way of looking at disease is that it is an invading force to be conquered. Another way is to approach disease as a difficult relationship that may be transformed into a healthy relationship. Each approach has its proper place. For example, a diabetic may prevent the damaging effects of the disease through diet and exercise. In this way, he transforms the relationship from a life threatening challenge to an opportunity for promoting a healthful lifestyle. This is a process of self-realization and adjustment of beliefs, attitudes and emotions. If you ignore diet and exercise, then a ripe environment for the disease may occur. Mind/body healing may shake a belief system to untangle limiting beliefs, or, work directly with emotions, or body energy, to change an unhealthy balance.

Life Energy

We tend to misunderstand the nature of a human being. We try to define the dynamics of the human system according to what we can observe, but the total human is beyond our understanding. The physical, emotional and intellectual aspects of being human have been studied extensively, but the subtle energy realm isn't as well defined. More complex electronic devices are being invented to measure and analyze the energetic nature of life. There are highly sophisticated EEGs, MRIs, CAT and PET scans, and more. Research shows we interact with other energy systems, as well. Experiments detect that the electromagnetic field around plants and even rocks changes as we approach them. Plants react with what we might call fear if we approach with the intent to cut off their stems, or leaves. The same plants relax when we approach to water them. The exercises throughout this E-book give you a feel for how this awareness works and how you can intentionally control your own life energy.

The body of universal energy (life energy) operates in a way that is similar to the universal water body that permeates all things within the earth's atmosphere, except that it is not confined to the earth. Energy by nature has no separation.

The movement of your life energy is a reflection of your intent in life. If you are an aggressive person you might puff your energy up in reptilian like display around your upper body in an effort to look bigger and more menacing. You see this in people who walk with elbows sticking out to claim as much space as possible. A person who has been abused may stay outside her body giving the appearance of no one being home. The physical and energy aspects are not separable. The energy manifests in the physical like a plant projecting an energetic outline of a leaf before it begins to grow the physical leaf. This energetic outline acts as a mold which is filled by the emerging leaf. The same dynamic works in a more complex human world as well. Every thought, movement, emotion and attitude is an envelope for delivering intent. Your intent is the mold that will be filled by your life energy.

You perform amazing feats with your soft body all the time but probably don't notice. You reach out with your soft body and connect to people, places, things and ideas and affect them with your energy, or intent. It's commonly believed that nothing moves faster than light but your mind can move faster. You can send your thought a million light years away in an instant. Spend time exploring the sensations in your heart and you will be amazed how you control aspects of your energy from here. Every part of your physical body is infused by your soft body in your own way. Each part of your body provides different ways to control, and interact with your soft body, and by extension, control and interact with the world around you. Put your awareness in various parts of your body and notice the quality of energy in each part, and how each part interacts with the outside world.

As you become more aware of your energetic nature, you will begin to notice the intent that allows your life challenges to exist. The form that your life challenges fill may have facets that include heredity, social conditioning, family dynamics, beliefs, emotions, spiritual relationships and physical attitudes. All of these are energetic events manifested in different ways. You can discover these aspects yourself through intent and awareness.

Energetic resource states can be used for healing. The works of Milton Erickson are full of references to using preexisting resource states. If you are working to heal a disease you might remember a time when you were strong and healthy. Notice how you held your energy in your body at this time. Consciously move the energy (awareness) in your body to match this healthy state. The more fully you focus your senses on the resource state the more you recreate the energetic aspects. Infuse your physical body with your life energy the same way you did when you were healthy. Notice the differences between how you held you energy then and how you hold it associated with the disease. Consciously adjust your energy to match the resource state as you go through your day and night. A variation is moving through your body with your awareness and finding places that seem to have too much energy concentrated there or too little. Move your energy around until it feels balanced. If it feels like you need a certain quality of energy, move that quality into the place that needs it. Trust your inner senses to guide you. Suspend beliefs that you lack the resources to heal, or to do anything else you choose.

The Soft Body

I adopted the name, soft body, to label our energetic aspect that experiences inside, and outside, our physical bodies. It moves wherever we send it, from the other side of the universe, to deep inside the molecules that make up our bodies. This is the part of us that animates our bodies, and leaves when we die. It responds perfectly, and instantly, to the movement of our awareness.

Your soft body does whatever you direct it to do. Your soft body, like your physical body, has capabilities we can't understand. You may have no idea how your muscles, joints, bones, and bio-chemistry work, but you can still walk. You walk because you have the ability to walk. You believe you can walk, and you kept trying until you learned to walk. Your soft bodies has abilities that you can discover and learn to use in your daily lives.

Researchers, under the direction of Robert O. Becker, M.D., measured the soft body under laboratory conditions. They found a constant low voltage direct current (DC) field that infuses the body. They found that the higher the concentration of energy, or consciousness, in the injured area, the quicker healing took place.

Directing and aiding healing is one way we can use our soft body awareness. Although it takes practice to learn, you don't have to strain. The soft body responds perfectly to your intent. As you use this energy for healing, you learn to use it in other areas of your life.

The study of physics tells us that all things are created from a universal energy. This universal energy is the essential building block of all things. Water, as it moves ceaselessly, never separating, is a good metaphor for the way universal energy infuses everything. Your body is almost entirely water. A certain amount of water moves through your body every day and must be replaced. You may be drinking water that was once consumed by a desert camel or by another human. The odds are that your body contains water molecules once consumed by Cleopatra, or any other being who lived more than 100 years ago.

The water in the moisture in your breath is connected to the vapor in the air, the water in and around the earth, and the water in your body. The water in your body, like the air you breath, is not something that you ever really own. Both are only yours to share as they pass through your body. Air and water are both like living bodies that are in constant change, shared by all living things while never separating from the larger body.

We share these life giving bodies with all things on earth, living and non-living. If it is true that all things are made entirely of essential energy, and this essential energy is pure consciousness, then the water, and the air, in your body has the potential to be aware of all water, and all air, everywhere through its connection with the universal bodies of water and air. In their ceaseless movement, water, and air, touch and pass through all things. This provides a universal connection with all things that contain water and air. With your soft body you can experience this same dynamic on a larger level. We all share the energy body of the universe.

Your Soft Body

This exercise introduces you to the soft body concept and helps increase awareness of what is going on inside. My approach to mind/body healing is to use my sensory awareness, inner and outer, as a connected unit or body. Awareness goes anywhere a person chooses to send it in any manner they choose.

Get comfortable and settle into your body. Noticing that each time you do this you become more aware of things, that you become more solid, more stable in the world. The more fully you settle into your body, the more solid and aware you become. There's an aspect of existence that when it is absent, our bodies become corpses. There are many names for this aspect. In this exercise we will call it the soft body. Bring your awareness to your feet and just notice how much of your feet you're aware of. Are your toes full of awareness? And how does your awareness fill your heels? The tops of your feet? Just notice how your consciousness fits in your feet. Do you fill your feet fully from heel to toe? From side-to-side? And top to bottom? And is this awareness of your soft body centered in your bones? How does it fit into your ankles? Is it aligned and centered there? Are you twisted or concentrated more in one side than the other? Are you concentrated more in the top or the bottom of your body? Just notice without judgment or the need to do anything about it.

And how is your awareness filling your lower legs at this moment? If your legs were vases and the awareness, the consciousness, or the soft body was water, how would that water fill your legs right now? Are there places that resist filling? Places where the awareness concentrates? Is your awareness centered in your bones? Are you twisted or more forward than backward or to either side in your legs? Are you long enough there? And how do you align from your knees to your hips? Are you centered and aligned in your bones? Are your upper legs full of awareness all the way to the skin? Does it move forward or backward? Is it too long or too short? Just notice. How do you align with your hips? Are they squared and centered? And is your pelvis full of awareness? Or are there places that don't seem to be aware, or places that are numb, or places you just can't put your awareness? Maybe there are places where the awareness is more concentrated, perhaps almost burning.

Notice how you're aligned with your spine. Do you have the full length of your spine? Are you centered with it? Is there any twisting pushing forward or backward zigzagging back and forth? Notice your torso. How do you infuse your torso with awareness? Are you aware of your inner organs? Are you aware of your heart beating, of the air moving in and out of your lungs, passing through your mouth and nose? Just notice how you fill your torso and where the awareness finds resistance.

Notice your fingers now. How do you align with the bones of your fingers and hands? Are you centered in the bones of your fingers, hands and wrists? How do you align with your lower arms? Just notice. From wrist to elbow to shoulder, how does your soft body awareness infuse your arms and shoulders?

And how does it fill your head? Do you infuse your entire brain with energy, or awareness, or only specific parts? And how vibrant are the senses that are centered in your head? Notice sight, sound, taste, smell, touch and the inner equivalents; the inner eye, the inner ear, the other senses. Take as much time as you choose to experience your soft body, and how it infuses your physical body. When you're ready, just let your eyes open naturally, and easily, and allow your consciousness to return to the room around you.

Vibrant Truth

Mind/body healing works with vibrant truths. Vibrant truth is when we use imaginary people, creatures, or things, along with real medicine and treatments. For example, the little boy mentioned earlier helped his brain tumor disappear by imagining white space ships that flew around and zapped the tumor with space rays. In reality this is totally inaccurate. Yet in its essence and results, it is true, accurate and effective. We have no white spaceships in our brains. But we have white blood cells, killer t-cells and macrophages that move through the blood and have the ability to annihilate tumors.

The Russians have done extensive research with biophotons. Biophotons are beams of light which each cell appears to emit on all measurable wavelengths. The space-type rays the boy used may be biophotons even though he did not know the actual working physiology of his immune system. He knew his immune system on an intuitive level and represented it to himself in images he could understand. His story was beyond the grasp of his doctors and beyond his knowledge to say what was actually happening.

It isn't important to understand how your body functions in a scientific, medical way. What is important is to bring your awareness to the problem and express your intent to heal on a level that you understand. Sometimes intellect can be the biggest barrier to effective action.

The Silent Witness

In cases of multiple personalities it is common for the different personalities to have different physical ailments. One personality may have allergies that disappear when another personality takes over. One personality may be diabetic while another in the same body is not. This supports the idea that mind, and body, are a whole unit and you can't change one without changing the other.

One personality, in cases of multiple personality disorder, often refers to itself as the one who was born with this body and the one who will continue after this body is laid down. This is the silent witness that retains consciousness during surgery or in a coma. Your silent witness is the part of you that is awake during sleep and the part that reaches out in the world to warn you of danger.

The presence of the silent witness is dramatically illustrated by two young boys, Roger and Jeff. Roger was three years old. He weighed less than one pound at birth. Doctors said he was no more than a vegetable. They thought him to be deaf, blind and without voluntary brain function. When I first met Roger it was on the pretext of doing therapeutic touch/unruffling in hopes he could go through a holiday season without pneumonia. I began to probe his soft body energy with my hands as I unruffled the energy layers. I gently cradled the back of his head in my hands as I connected heart to heart with him. I felt a flash of emotion as he and I made contact between our silent witnesses. Roger began to cry, something he hadn't done before unless he was in extreme physical pain. This time it seemed as if he noticed other life existed for the first time and he wasn't alone. His cries seemed a mixture of joy, sadness, hope and loneliness. Since then Roger is more aware of his family, and they feel he knows they are around. He also made it through the holidays without pneumonia for the first time and continues to grow healthier. He attends a special school where he seems to enjoy being in the circle when games are being played. He responds to the touch and presence of other children.

The other boy, Jeff, was about ten and facing two long, difficult back operations to install steel rods along his spine. Before the surgeries, we spent only a short time together. What seemed most important and potentially dangerous, as I understood it, was the extreme blood loss that might occur. We focused most of our time on him learning to stay partially conscious, and monitor the amount of blood lost. I suggested some different ways Jeff might control the blood loss and keep the area where the surgery was taking place free of blood that might hinder the progress of the operations. I suggested he could draw the blood away from the operations by imagining it being blocked from getting to the area. He used images of his blood vessels constricting to squeeze off the blood flow, his heart beating slower and his body becoming colder.

I suggested that his silent witness could be aware of the operations to watch for complications to prevent them before they happened. I offered these suggestions to Jeff while he was in a deep hypnotic state. After the actual operations the surgeon said that they were the best surgeries he had ever done. He said it was as if something, or someone, had been guiding him. The blood loss during both operations was about half the amount predicted.

In both boys, it seems as if they contacted some greater aspect and this greater aspect began to take an active role in their healing.

Awareness and Intent

I knew a cat named Spunky. Spunky had bladder problems caused by seafood. Crystals formed in his bladder and clogged it so much he couldn't urinate. He came close to death several times before he (the cat) learned how to manage his problem including adjusting what he ate and the person who fed him. The first time he got sick the veterinarian prescribed pills to keep the crystals from forming. Spunky hated pills. He was an amiable cat in most situations, unless he was being given medicine, then he had to be wrapped in a towel to control him long enough to administer his pill. He became very good at pretending to swallow the pill, but it would be found later on the floor or under the couch. When he took his pills every day he was all right.

Spunky learned quickly that seafood caused his problems and simply quit eating it. With this awareness came a natural intent that led him to take the right action to solve his bladder problem and keep him alive. But that wasn't enough. He still got sick.

Spunky was a well behaved cat who seldom jumped on counters or begged. Most of the time he was tolerant and dignified. Suddenly, however, he began jumping on the counter or the table. This was puzzling since he was not usually eager to eat. He persisted until he got what he needed to dissolve the crystals. Asparagus! It took him only a few days to train his person to prepare three asparagus spears for him every day. He never let her forget and he had no more bladder problems for the rest of his life.

The intelligence essential for knowing a life challenge is very primitive. Spunky discovered his life challenge, found what caused it and came up with a solution. His intent was to heal himself. He didn't want to die. He gained guidance from the life challenge and took corrective action based on this guidance. The difference between Spunky and a human with a similar condition is that Spunky lacked an emotional agenda or limiting beliefs to attach to his life challenge. He simply chose to live and proceeded to survive and thrive. As people, we have hidden and unconscious conditioning that we bring to healing. There are usually secondary gains in being sick such as knowing we only get the touching and intimacy we need when sick. Old beliefs set limits like: My mother, grandmother and great-grandmother had gallstones and I will get them; or cancer is incurable and even if I survived I would always be in pain anyway. These are underlying emotional stressors that cause a continuous low level panic. When you focus on a life challenge address all the aspects you discover as you discover them having faith in your innate mind/body intelligence to present them at the right time and in the most productive order. Be open to seeing your limiting beliefs and adjusting them.

Awareness and intent are the essential dynamics in all human creation. We intend that something happens in our world and in the act of intending we cause awareness that leads to actions to reach our goals. If we follow this guidance by taking the right action, we can reach our reasonable goals. A reasonable goal is one that fits within the boundaries of our belief system. If the goal you require in your life is not within your belief system you can adjust your beliefs through new learning and understanding, verbal and nonverbal.

Cybernetics, the study of electromechanical control systems, describes the physical process of producing an outcome such as grasping a glass of water. We make many adjustments until the glass is in hand. This is an unconscious process that happens with such speed that we can't think of or be aware of every movement. Imagine how difficult it would be to get a drink of water if you had to think through each step of the process. How long would it take you to bring your awareness to and coordinate each muscle along with interactions with other muscles, nerves and body systems to make each tiny adjustment required to reach, grasp and drink. These adjustments are automatic in practice.

Psycho Cybernetics is the same process of adjustment on a psychological level. Most actions in life can be compared to piloting a sailboat. While under sail, the boat is off course more than ninety percent of the time. The pilot makes many minor adjustments to arrive at his destination. If he makes no adjustments, he won't arrive at his planned destination.

If you intend an outcome and you bring your awareness to the situation, you will automatically find guidance inside and outside yourself. If you take the action directed by your awareness, you will eventually reach your goal. You will reach your destination even if you start going in the wrong direction as long as you continue to make adjustments along the way. Even mistakes move you ever closer to your goal. If you don't take the appropriate action, you may not reach your goal. Like sailing a boat, this requires constant adjustments directed the guidance of your sensory feedback.

Some corrective action is automatic. If you put your hand on something hot, you immediately pull your hand away without thinking. Nothing told you verbally to move your hand, but there was a guidance to move it. Your sensory feedback (awareness) provides the guidance to adjust your actions (intent) to create your desired outcome.

Your ability to effectively follow your inner guidance can be inhibited by your limiting beliefs. If you believe you cannot heal a life challenge, then your intent to heal is limited by that belief. You will inhibit your healing and be blind to your inner guidance.

Healing is a personal thing. You define healing in your way. One person with cancer might find that healing for him is complete remission with no scars. Another person's healing might be to accept himself and the things he did during his lifetime before he dies. Only you can know what healing means to you.

Healing on a personal level moves you toward a life that fulfills you as a person, regardless of what form that takes. At the end of your life you will die like everyone else. When you have reached the end of this life's journey, the only real healing is to let go of your body to continue your journey. All great mystics, healers and gurus die. Most die from the same causes as people in general. Some die in extreme pain from cancer although, they may have a different relationship with pain and cancer than most people. They may savor the wonder of living and embrace each moment in a celebration of life accepting the pain as part of the gift of life.

Awareness and intent are key to all mind/body healing techniques. The simplest and most direct technique in directing one's own healing is to simply bring awareness to your life challenge with the intent to heal. If you only wish a thing without taking action you probably won't get results. Working with your awareness is taking action.

Stress may be a source of growth or regression depending on how you react to it. We can choose how to understand and interact with the world inside and outside ourselves and we have the ability to choose our attitude in any situation making our stress strengthening or weakening.

We have the capacity to change simply by intending change to happen and taking action to move toward it. In the 1960's, Fritz Perls said that awareness is curative in itself. Ron Kurtz wrote about organicity or the innate capacity of all life to heal itself. Kurtz believes people have the capacities necessary to heal any given problem, discomfort or disease according to what is appropriate to their healing. If you intend to heal, your awareness begins to bring into your consciousness the necessary action to cause that healing. The intent guides the awareness that guides the intent. It is a self-perpetuating cycle that continues until the goal is reached or abandoned.

Grounding

The first step in becoming more aware of and consciously directing your own subtle energy work is to increase your presence. Presence is simply being here with no thoughts of the past or future, just attending to now with all your senses. Complete presence is a feat seldom achieved.

The easiest, quickest and most readily learned method of increasing presence is grounding. Grounding helps you become more aware of your body. Emotional content may emerge as you become more present. The pain you feel in your body may be emotional in origin as often as it is physical. If you bring your awareness to the pain, the emotional aspects may become apparent to you. The following brief exercise helps develop deeper awareness of your body in a safe way.

As you go through the following grounding exercise notice how your sensual acuity changes as you become more grounded. Notice how grounding affects your feeling of safety and well-being. Notice how it affects your sense of time.

I invite you to sit upright with your feet flat on the floor. Take three deep breaths and begin to settle in your body. Notice where you are right now. How much of your body are you aware of? Just notice without the need to do anything, without judgment. Just notice where you are at. Bring your awareness to the bottoms of your feet. How aware of your feet are you right now? Bring more awareness into your feet. Bring more awareness to the soles of your feet. Let every cell become alive and aware all the way from the tips of your toes to your heels and the pads of your toes. Now feel the curls of your toes and the balls of your feet and your arches. Feel your heels, the outside edges of your feet then your entire foot at once. Notice now that with the bottoms of your feet you can feel whatever they are resting on. If you are wearing socks, notice that you can feel the material of your socks and you can feel the weave of the material. You can let that feeling move a little deeper.

If you're wearing shoes, you can feel the soles of your shoes. You can feel the way they're made and the materials that they're made of. You can let your feeling move a little deeper going out a little farther you can feel the floor, perhaps it's carpeted. Perhaps it's wood or tile. Whatever it is, just notice that it feels different from the soles of your shoes and your socks. Let your awareness reach into it like roots, going deeper, spreading out farther. Let your feeling move down to whatever is beneath the top layer of the floor.

Perhaps it's wood or concrete. Just notice that it feels different. It feels more stable, more secure. Let your roots go deeper, now, right through the building you're in, perhaps moving through a basement or through many floors. Just let your roots keep going until they reach into the earth. Notice that you can feel the texture of the earth beneath the building. You can feel the coolness and the darkness. You can feel the moisture. Let your roots go as deep as you choose, even all the way through the earth if that feels right.

Roots have two purposes; one is for strength and stability and the other is to bring back nourishment and information. Experience the way things are different as you ground. Notice the quality of your senses and your degree of serenity. Take as much time as you choose to explore how things change when you ground.

Grounding II

This grounding exercise is from Tai Chi and reveals some benefits of being grounded. This exercise requires two people. Person #1 stands relaxed with a normal state of mind. Person #2 gently pushes #1's shoulder until he is pushed off balance. The first person now imagines dense roots growing deep into the earth from his feet and the second person pushes again. Both now feel that person #1 is more solid and harder to push off balance. Repeat the sequence only this time, person #1 fills his legs and pelvis with awareness along with the roots from his feet. His stability again increases. Repeat several times and then switch roles with your partner.

Grounding to the Opposite

Sit comfortably with your back straight and settle into your body. Begin to bring your soft body into alignment with your physical body. When you are sufficiently grounded, centered and present, begin to probe your body with your awareness. Notice that within your body there are many different feelings. You may find tension and relaxation. You may find pain and pleasure. You may find within your body the opposite of any feeling you find present. Within us exists the potential for all things. If you find joy inside, sorrow must be within as well. If you find pain, there must be the potential for ecstasy. They cannot exist separately.

Bring your awareness to your life challenge and experience the feelings, images, sounds, words, colors or whatever you find. You can trust anything that you find is exactly the right experience for the moment.

Find an area of your body that has the opposite experience and connect the two places with energy. You may connect the areas with breath, color, light, sound, vibration or any other energy form to enhance the connection. Try whatever feels right for you. You can always adjust it or quit using it if it doesn't help.

For example, if you find a burning pain inside, you can scan your body until you find a place of coolness. The opposite is always there. Connect the place of coolness to the area of the burning pain. You may feel the urge to imagine a cool blue light connecting the places. Let these places blend. As a client said, "It's like introducing it (life challenge) to another part of the body so it can teach it how to be healthy."

Mindfulness

Grounding helps establish a state of mind known as mindfulness, or presence. Mindfulness is a state of being aware with all your senses. You observe in an impersonal way without judgment or the need to take any action. See through the eyes of the one inside who sees through your eyes. Listen to the one who listens inside. It is the silent reporter position. A good reporter reports the observable facts without interjecting his own judgment or interfering.

Wu Wei

Another useful attitude when doing these exercises is wu wei. Wu wei (pronounced woo-way) is a Taoist term for moving through life with ease. Wu wei is the art of being present with each moment of your life without the constant chatter of the inner voices. The practices of Zen, Yoga, Taoism and martial arts all use exercises for developing inner silence and presence. When practicing wu wei, you meet each moment of life with no attitude, no judgment and a demeanor of inner silence. Wu wei is like flowing water, always adjusting to more with the least resistance toward its goal.

If your house falls down, you simply begin to rebuild. In any situation, no matter how drastic, you take the correct action, wasting no energy. This doesn't mean you deny your feelings. It means you feel more fully, having no judgments about yourself or what you feel. It is a matter of walking the earth with practical feet.

The key attitudes emphasized throughout the rest of this eBook are presence, mindfulness, being grounded and mercy for yourself – the opposite of self-judgment.

Where Is the Center of Your Universe?

Sit erect with your feet on the floor and take a deep breath. Settle into your body and become more grounded. With your eyes closed, bring your awareness to one inch in front of your spine. Notice where this awareness is in relation to your physical spine. The location of this awareness changes from moment to moment. Sometimes it is even outside your physical body.

Make a mental picture of the world around you. Notice if more of your world is in front of you or behind you. Notice if you sense more world existing to your left or to your right. Notice if more of your world is above you or below you. Do you exist at the center of your world or have you placed yourself off center? Are you more to the front, back, either side, above or below or a combination of any of the above? Notice if you exist more inside or outside your body. Which is larger, inside or outside? Notice where you place yourself in your world while going through your daily life.

We All Share the Same Water

Our bodies are mainly water. It's something we share with most living beings. We humans come and go on this Earth but the water that allows our bodies to live stays. Even while we live the water in our bodies constantly cycle through to be replaced by fresh water. The water in our bodies constantly moves outward through sweat and other elimination processes always an unconnected part of the larger of body water that permeated and surrounds the Earth. At the same time it moves inward from food and drink to passing through our personal water bodies. It is a continual process that connects all the water in our bodies with all the water leaving and entering our bodies.

The same is true for the other living beings on this planet. The water that moves through our bodies without disconnection or interruption is connected to the Earth's water body and to all the water contained in all the living and non-living water containing things on the planet. There is no separation of the water in our bodies and the water in others. The same is true of the air we breathe. It constantly cycles through all things that contain air without separation. The air you just inhaled is part of a single body of air we all share.

Your soft body is like the water and air that your physical body contain. It has the illusion of being separate from the total pool of essential energy, yet, it is not separate. It is not possible to separate yourself from the universal energy. Your body provides the means to experience not only your personal life energy but any part of the universal energy as well. There is no separation.

The Eagle

This is an especially energizing and uplifting exercise.

Settle into your body and center yourself inside your body. Notice what's going on inside right now. Begin to follow your breath inward, breathing deeper with each breath. Move your breath deeper into your body and farther back with each breath. Imagine a tap root beginning at the base of your skull, following your spine downward, out your tail bone, deep into the earth, reaching all the way to the molten center of the earth. Send anything that is appropriate to let go of at this time to the earth's core to be vaporized by the intense heat. You might choose to release attitudes or beliefs that don't serve you. You might choose to release toxicity of any sort spiritual, emotional or physical. Release whatever you find into the core of the earth, pushing it downward with each breath until it has all been incinerated.

Imagine that at the very tip of your tap root at the core of the earth is a vibration, like the buzzing of a bumble bee flapping its wings. Notice that you can feel that same buzzing and flapping at the end of your tail bone. Allow that vibration to expand like a hummingbird flapping its wings at your tail bone. Let it amplify even more as if it were a larger bird. The wings of this bird tickle the insides of your hips as it flaps and begins to rise, slowly moving up toward your chest, massaging all that it touches with awareness, bringing it to life. It flies right out through the center of your chest and way off in the distance you see an eagle. A huge magnificent eagle, floating on the air currents, soaring high above the ground, feathers rippling in the wind. The eagle is able to see a blade of grass a mile below and see and feel the sound of the earth itself, the song of the mountains and oceans even though they may be thousands of mile away.

Each time the eagle's wings rise there is a gentle tugging at the center your chest, in your heart area. Each time they rise, you feel the strength of those magnificent wings gently and lovingly pulling at your heart. As the wings fall there's a release in your heart. Rise and pull, fall and release. Rise and pull, fall and release. The eagle flies toward you. As it flies close enough you can see, and even feel, the details of the feathers, the beak and the talons. Suddenly, it transforms into a sphere of spinning light. The light in the sphere is the exact same color as the light in your heart. You realize that this is part of your heart. It has always been a part of your heart. As it moves closer, you choose to open yourself to allow the sphere to return to your heart where it belongs. Let it merge. Experience whatever you experience without judgment. Notice what you're feeling and what you're knowing. Take all the time you need or want. When you're ready, just allow your eyes to open and your consciousness to return to the room around you.

Boundaries

The term boundaries is common but the nature of boundaries is usually only defined in terms of the negative results of having poor boundaries. We speak of boundaries in terms of lack of boundaries, enmeshment or failure to separate ourselves from others. We see the dynamics of poor boundaries in depression and schizophrenia, but we seldom realize our own boundaries. The natural action of mirror neurons cause us to connect with other people, and maybe other animals, can make this difficult. Experiencing your energetic boundaries and your energetic relationships with other people is essential to recognizing the influence of other people on you and your health as well as your subtle influences on them. Therapists often ask their clients to develop good boundaries without giving them a working definition of what a boundary is, let alone differences between a good boundary and a poor boundary. Some simple exercises used to increase awareness of boundaries are presented here.

Perceiving Body Energy

The following two-person exercises come from the practice of therapeutic touch and will help you develop awareness of your life energy using your own senses.

Take a few moments to become grounded. Have one person lie down. Move about ten to twelve feet from this person. With your hand open and your palm pointed toward the person, slowly move your hand closer. As you come closer, notice any sensations you feel in your palm. You may feel warmth or cold. You may feel a vibration or roughness. There are many sensations you might feel. Whatever you feel is right. Therapeutic touch practitioners say that there are seven layers of subtle sensations (energy layers) that you may feel as you continue to approach until you touch the other person. Notice how many layers you feel. It is unlikely that you can feel all seven layers the first time you try this. It takes practice to develop this sensitivity.

If you are the person lying down, notice how it feels to be approached this way. How is it different with your eyes closed? How does it feel to have someone move through the energy layers?

If possible, have a different person lie down now and notice the differences in the feel of the energy field between the two. Use several more people, if available, and note any similarities or differences among them.

Registered nurses practice therapeutic touch in hospitals aid in the treatment of various health problems. Therapeutic touch is easy to learn. An adult family member can learn to take over treatment in a few hours. Using energy to aid in healing is a powerful technique that anyone can learn.

In the practice of modern medicine doctors measure human energy fields in many ways in the diagnosis of disease and injury. Some are EKG, MRI, EEG, CAT and PET scans. We cannot dispute these energy fields or that they reflect certain health facts about individuals. We already know that people can feel and use this energy. How does this affect our daily lives? An exercise to explore this from Ron Kurtz's Body-Centered Psychotherapy, The Hakomi Method follows.

The Power of Touch

Do this exercise with two people. Start by settling into your body and bringing your awareness into the present. One person, the receiver, sits in a comfortable position noticing what she feels in her body. The other person, the giver, waits until the first person is ready then begins to move her hand very slowly, with palm open, toward the other person. Both people note the automatic reactions occurring within their minds and bodies as the hand approaches to touch a prearranged spot on the receiver's body. Perhaps, touch the person's shoulder or face. Ask where he or she wants to be touched. The giver allows the touch to linger, with palm open, resting gently on the receiver for about ten seconds and then very slowly moves the hand away. Both people should notice anything, no matter how subtle, that happens as the touch lingers and then as the hand is removed. Talk about your experience while it's happening. Pause at any point to listen to your partner's experience, but stay on track. Keep conversation focused on what you are experiencing first hand, right now. Repeat the above sequence and then reverse roles. If you in the role of receiver feel any discomfort from the approaching hand, hold the wrist and guide the approaching hand. By guiding the hand, this gives you the power to stop the touch at any point. With touch, safety is of supreme importance.

Next, both partners take time to ground and connect heart to heart. Each person reaches out with the feeling from her heart and connects to the other person each allowing the other into her heart. Repeat the exercise with the heart to heart connection and notice any difference.

You will probably experience some emotion during the preceding exercise. This may be anything from a slight feeling of contentment or anxiety to catharsis or extreme fear. This exercise shows the touch that causes the most profound reaction in us isn't always the physical touch. Once we enter the boundaries of the energy field of another person, it seems that we cause a reaction in that person and in ourselves. Let's explore how far away we have to be to cause a reaction in another person with another exercise from Ron Kurtz.

When Does a Touch Begin?

This exercise is to be done in pairs. Both partners settle into their bodies and bring their awareness to the present. One person stands against a wall with eyes closed while the other approaches silently from a distance of at least twenty feet. Use a longer approach if possible. The receiving person will raise her hand each time she would like the approaching person to stop, allowing the receiver more time to feel the sensations. The approaching person then stops until the receiving person drops her arm. The approaching person continues until he is only a few inches from the receiver. The receiver then opens her eyes to check the distance between the two. The receiver closes her eyes again while the approaching person slowly and silently backs away to his original position.

Change roles and repeat the process. Try different variations like one person walking toward two or three others, or two people walking simultaneously toward one person. Approach from the side or back of the first person. Notice the different ways this exercise affects you emotionally and how it affects your sense of well-being and feeling of safety. Notice the distance from which you can feel another or be felt by them and the way that your approach affects others. Sense the quality of your feelings and any other aspect that may interest you.

Repeat the preceding exercises. This time, the approaching person chooses a situation or incident that evokes strong emotion. He holds these images in his mind as he again approaches. Notice any difference in your experience.

Next the approached person imagines all her life energy being drawn into an imaginary egg shell surrounding and protecting her body. Now approach while experiencing strong emotion and notice any difference in the experience. This is a quick and easy way to experience and learn to work with your boundaries.

You have probably experienced that your awareness extends some distance from your body and interacts with others. Grounding and centering (as experienced in the soft body exercise) and bringing your energy tightly around you like a protective egg help to create and maintain distinct boundaries and make you aware when you are being affected by others.

Unruffling

The following exercise from therapeutic touch helps you become more intimately aware of the energy aspects of your body. You also may learn to be aware of more of the subtleties of your life. This practice is called unruffling and is the most basic and easiest to learn energy healing technique.

Begin by grounding. The person doing the unruffling imagines an invisible connection between his heart and the heart of the receiver. This is a very important step. It increases the sensory and energetic bonds that develop between the giver and the receiver and helps the giver become more sensitive to the subtle physical and energetic shifts in the receiver. The intent of the unruffler also is very important. The heart to heart connection helps to keep the intent of the procedure clear and provides safety for the receiver.

The receiver lies down. The giver slowly moves his palm toward the receiver's body from a distance of eight to ten feet. Note any changes in the feel of space surrounding the receiver with your palm as you approach. At a distance of six to twelve inches probe the space surrounding the receiver. Notice anything that registers in your senses, inner and outer, as different or changing in any perceivable quality, keeping your hands moving at a slow steady pace. Moving them too slow or too fast or stopping decreases the sensitivity of your palms. You may sense heat or cold, tingling or soothing, rough or bumpy or other sensations not necessarily limited to tactile feel.

You don't have to search for a right feeling. Any area that feels different from the surrounding area is an appropriate place to work. An area of different feeling usually relates to injury, imbalance or disease in the physical body. If the receiver is uncomfortable or in pain, the area above the discomfort is a likely to feel different from surrounding areas. Let your hands guide themselves by feel to the proper distance from the body to work. Now, begin to stroke, or smooth, the energy above the area. Continue to smooth the energy layer until it feels the same as the surrounding areas. In practice you might move from one area to another until the entire area around the body feels consistent. You may unruffle a single area or you may continue working until the entire body is balanced at all levels you are able to sense.

When working on yourself, you may use the hands of your soft body to unruffle, massage or balance any area of your body. If you have tension in your back, close your eyes and settle into your body. Imagine yourself standing behind yourself massaging your back in the exact right spot and in exactly the right way. If you have a deep muscle pain or cramp, imagine reaching inside the muscle with your soft body hands and massaging it. The soft body isn't limited to the surface of your body. You can massage internal organs or between layers of muscles. You can use your soft body in any way your imagination allows. When using this technique, it may be helpful to use imagery or sound. See in your mind's eye what your hands feel. Send sound through your hands to help repair, balance, clean, soothe or deliver any other intention. Use any method you choose to deliver healing intent, the more fun the better. Using your soft body to rehearse anything you want to learn or become better at will accelerate your mastery of whatever it is, including healing yourself or others.

Healing Water

This exercise in energy healing might surprise you with your own abilities as an energy healer. Try working with something small, like indigestion, to start. Water is an amazing substance for holding and transferring energy. Have a glass of water ready for this exercise. Distilled water is best, but tap water will do.

Settle into your body and bring more feeling to the palms of your hands. Hold your hands, palms facing, about 3-4" apart, moving your right hand slowly, clockwise over your left palm. Feel a warmth begin to develop.

Bring to mind the life challenge that you are working on as you continue moving your right hand over your left, letting the warmth build as if you were rolling a ball of heat between your hands. Remember a time your life challenge didn't exist. If has existed as long as you can remember, bring an image to mind of a person who doesn't face your challenge. Use an image of this person's health as a resource state. Put the feeling of health into the ball of heat you are rolling in your hands. Intensify it. Make it denser and hotter. When you're ready, put that ball of energy into your glass of water. Drink it and notice how you feel. You can use this technique for any life challenge, physical or non-physical.

Expansion and Contraction Exercise

Settle into your body and begin to experience your skin. Fill your body with awareness all the way to your skin. Begin to bring your awareness into your torso, making it smaller. Let your awareness move down just into your heart, becoming the size of your heart. Now, let your awareness shrink to the size of a golf ball, to the size of a marble, to the size of a pea. Continuing on down to the size of a single cell, shrinking smaller and smaller to the size of an atom. And now shrinking to the size of a subatomic particle, smaller than the smallest particle that makes up matter. Shrinking to half that size and half that size again.

Now allow your awareness to grow larger, to the size of a subatomic particle. To the size of an atom and growing to the size of a single cell, a pea, a marble, a golf ball, the size of your heart. The size of your body, the size of the room you're in, the size of the building you're in, growing to the size of the town you're in. And continuing to grow to the size of the state or country you are in and growing to the size of your continent, the size of your hemisphere, to the size of the earth, filling the earth's skin perfectly as if it were your own. Growing large enough now to include the moon and growing to the size of our solar system, to the size of our galaxy, the size of our galaxy cluster, growing to the size of the universe and to size of all that exists and just a little bit bigger.

Now begin to grow smaller to the size of the universe. shrink to the size of our galaxy cluster, to the size of the milky way, to the size of our solar system, to the size of the earth, growing to the size of your hemisphere bringing your awareness back to the size of your continent, back to the size of your country, to the size of your town, to the size of the building you are in and growing back to the size of your skin. Filling your skin perfectly and fully.

Take all the time you choose to feel what you may be experiencing. When you're ready allow your eyes to open and your consciousness to return to the room around you.

CHAPTER 3
FOUR REALMS OF HEALING

Four realms that may be used in mind/body healing are: spiritual, emotional, intellectual and physical. All are aspects of the energy continuum as it vibrates at different rates from pure energy to physical manifestation.

The easiest path to exploring your life challenge is starting at the sensations in your body and following them through the realms of emotion, belief and energy (or spiritual) to the place where they begin. When changing your relationships with your life challenge, it's easier to work in the other direction. Changes made on an energetic level will affect all other levels. If resistance to these changes exists on the emotional, belief or physical levels, it may be proper to work on those levels as well. It's easier to change an emotional charge by altering the belief that supports it than to change it by relieving its bodily symptoms. Beliefs change automatically when supporting intention or attitude change. It's possible to change the emotional charge by working with the physical symptoms, but it's more efficient to work with supporting beliefs and/or unresolved traumas.

The sensations in your physical body create a map. Your beliefs fill in the details. The emotion reveal the intent. Your relationship with the world outside yourself influences all of these. These can be discovered through the feelings in your body and changed by choosing change and following through with effective action from the guidance of your own awareness.

Relationship

All aspects of the following realms of healing can be expressed as relationships. All aspects of your being are reflected by your relationships: interpersonal and intrapersonal.

Your soft body is pure energy potential that molds itself as defined by the influences and possibilities within your DNA, environment and psychological makeup. Intent determines which possibilities will be expressed and which will not. Studies indicate that meditation can change the way we express our DNA by turning on and off genes and changing the intensity of the expression of genes. I have a 65% genetic chance of expressing obesity but I have never been obese. Another way of saying this is that intent is the choice of what will be infused with life energy (soft body) and what will not be infused. You can consciously influence how your DNA is expressed by your intent as an individual. Just because you have a dark, icky color in your palate doesn't mean that it will tint everything in your life. Dark, icky colors are great for shadows. As a developing embryo you had the potential for expressing as any form of life on earth. Yet, you developed as a human expressing yourself with human features as opposed to flippers and hooves. This is the biological intent of our species.

Your relationships with yourself and others influence the way you infuse your body with energy. A respectful, loving relationship may allow you to infuse your body with ease, joy and wonder. A relationship of anger may cause you to restrict energy flow in your body or cause it to stagnate in certain areas. Other relationships may cause you to lose or withdraw all but essential life energy from your body as a defense against fear or pain. All these things alter the flow of energy through your brain and your body. Some are sources of chronic stress.

As humans, we are sensitive to the emotional charges of those around us. A metaphor for this is a tuning fork. If you strike one tuning fork and bring it close to another tuning fork of the same frequency the second fork will begin to vibrate, even if it is of another octave. If you strike a C fork and bring it next to a C fork that is an octave higher or lower, it will still vibrate. This is called resonance. If you bring the same C fork next to a fork of any other frequency, even one only slightly different from C, the second fork won't vibrate. It doesn't resonate.

We have mirror neurons that cause us to empathize with others by feeling what they feel at a very intimate level. Researchers discovered that monkeys' brains reacted the same when they performed a task as when they observed the task. Their brains acted in unison with the researcher's brains. We have the same capacity along with the ability to turn it on or off. We empathize with those we feel are like us more easily than those we think are different.

Emotions resonate in a similar way. For example, if someone you work with is yelled at by the boss, she may feel anger and shame. As a fellow human you will feel her anger and shame to the degree that you empathize with your co-worker. If the person is your friend, you will more intensely feel her anger and shame than if she is someone you don't like. Regardless of who it is, even if you don't know her or know that she was yelled at, you will resonate with her to some extent feeling some anger and shame. If the boss is more like you, in your mind, you will feel the bosses fear, anger and frustration bringing back memories associated with these feelings. As a matter of mental health, we develop defense mechanisms to lessen our resonance with others. Those who lose the ability to muffle the resonance tend to end up in mental institutions.

Recently, I demonstrated resonance to a college class. During the demonstration, a student started crying as she talked about a family member with cancer. Suddenly, she jumped up and ran from the room. Everyone in the room felt her intense emotion. Another student asked, "Is that what you mean by resonance?"

"Yes," I affirmed.

This opportune moment could have been used more fully if I had pointed out that all of us in the room had common reactions in our bodies. I could have pointed out that our breathing had moved to our upper chests while our bellies tightened. I might have brought awareness to the tightening each of us felt in our throats or the buildup of soft body energy in our chests. I might have had students notice whether memories of personal tragedies were streaming into their awareness. In the moment, I was resonating with her sorrow and fear. Like the others in the class, I felt like crying and missed the opportunity.

Imagine living in an environment where everyone around you is always angry. With anger, there is always fear. Anger and its supporting fear are common conditions in many families. If you live your life in anger, your body will bear the consequences of constant stress. Anger tightens your jaw and neck. It concentrates soft body energy in your head where your angry thoughts run. Your shoulders and back tighten and your heart rate and blood pressure increase while your breathing becomes restricted. Fight or flight hormones course through your body. When you walk into a room, everyone's neck and jaw tightens. They unconsciously react with defensive strategies like attacking you, getting away from you or ignoring you. This creates an internal environment that may result in any number of health consequences for you and those around you.

Some people claim that you create your world and your life challenge. It is true that how you experience the world must fit into your belief system. Your world tends to stay consistent with your constant narration of your experience. When you resonate unchecked with the people around you, your thoughts and feelings are subject to the whims of anyone who comes near. When you are aware of this, you can choose to control your resonance with others.

Relationships in healing can be helpful or harmful. I attended the first annual AIDS, Medicine and Miracles conference many years ago. Like most of the world at that time, I thought that all people who were HIV-positive developed full-blown AIDS and died within a year. I was very afraid, not only because of my fear of getting AIDS by contact, but because of my homophobic feelings I didn't believe I had before I got out of my car and found I was afraid to go into the building.

I had never heard of long-term survivors, but at the conference there were some who had survived for as long as ten years. Many of the survivors seemed healthy. The thing that became clear as each long-term survivor spoke was that each one knew why they had survived. They had no doubt about it. They knew they had survived because they were in solid, supportive, loving relationships. They spoke about their mates using the same words that I might use to describe a loving relationship. This went a long way toward healing my fear of homosexuals as I resonated with their celebration of their loving relationships. My attitudes changed and my beliefs followed.

Intent is the choice of which potential reality you will adopt. Intent is expressed in many ways. Every action, physical posture, emotional attitude, spoken word, internal dialogue, visualization, breath dynamic, sound expressed internally or externally and an infinite number other aspects of life express your intent.

Underlying all intent is belief. When you embrace opposing beliefs the resulting stress may create health problems that can manifest on any level including physical, intellectual, emotional and spiritual.

This example of a family in therapy illustrates this interplay of belief and intent and how it affects health. A man took his wife for an emergency therapy session. She had just undergone a double mastectomy as the result of breast cancer. She was told that her chances of survival for six weeks was about 35 percent. She agreed to the session to appease her husband's demands. It was immediately apparent that she was the heart of the family. The family included a teenage son, a married daughter in her early twenties, the daughter's husband and an infant child. The woman was very clear in the belief that she was dying because her family was falling apart.

The whole family was brought in to be involved in the healing process. The children put up heavy resistance at first. The husband had been extremely domineering and was described as a tyrant. He agreed that this had been the case in the past, but assured his family that he was willing to change in order to help his wife survive. The family members were suspicious but agreed to at least try to help their mother choose to live. She had stated clearly that she intended to die if her family could not come together and act like a family.

After bringing the family together, the mother began to make some progress in healing. She responded to the stated intent of the family to begin to work out their differences. The turning point in her healing process came a few weeks later. Her husband almost dragged her into a session. She had decided that her family wasn't sincere in their efforts to become a functional family. She stated that she wasn't going to do anything to survive. She was committed to dying.

She sat defiantly, daring anyone to try to talk her out of dying as soon as possible. She and her husband were both shocked when she was encouraged to do what she believed was best. She was assured that if she chose death, she would be supported. Work began to help her prepare herself to die in a loving way, leaving no unfinished business behind. Her sobbing husband was assured that if she chose death, there was nothing anyone could do but support her in her resolve. Death is the ultimate and appropriate end to life. When you die, it should be with the loving support of your friends and family. The result of this session was that she chose life. Her husband chose to honestly work with her and the children to create a healthy family. The children were still suspicious, but were willing to find and work with their own therapists after their father admitted to the many crimes he had committed against them and their mother. The family confessed its deepest secrets. They claimed responsibility as the offenders and the healing process began in earnest for the mother, each family member and the family as a unit. As the family healed, so did the mother, despite her refusal to give up smoking and drinking. Six months later, her oncologist informed her that she was in remission. A year and a half later, at last report, she was very healthy, in complete remission and still smoking and drinking.

Her family was healing. All violence stopped after the children found that they could confront their parents with perceived offenses that were committed against them in the past without fear of retaliation. The children were willing to truly cooperate after they found that no matter how far or how hard they pushed their father, he would no longer strike out at them or act in a tyrannical manner. Each family member gained self-respect and self-esteem. They had reason to survive as a family and their mother had reason to survive.

The husband's intent in this example is equally important in his wife's healing process. He admitted to being manipulative and demanding control over the family. This reflected his belief that he had the right and duty to be in control of his family. Not being in control meant that he was a failure as a man, a father and a husband. He believed he had the right to use violence to maintain his dominance.

A country western ballad called, "*Daddy*", constantly went through his mind. This ballad was about a man who died and was seen as tough but fair by his surviving children. He was seen as a tyrant. This song constantly reaffirmed his beliefs about the nature of being a man and fueled his intent to continue his strategy toward his family. Although, he promised to change, his real intent was to continue his tyranny. He believed he would be able to force his wife and children to live up to his expectations until his wife made him realize that he was not in control. In fact, he never had been in control.

When she demonstrated to him that she could die without his consent, his world was upset. The inconsistency in his beliefs and what was happening in the world caused panic attacks that required hospitalization. During the family healing process, he felt helpless at first. His panic attacks revealed his intent that someone fix his life for him. Underlying this intent was the belief that he was unable to do anything to affect his own healing, but someone else could do it for him. It also revealed the belief that he was right all along and had no reason to change. His healing began when he admitted to himself and his family that he had never intended to change before. Now that the stakes were his wife's life, he finally gave in and worked to change in earnest. His willingness to change removed one more barrier to his wife's healing process.

His promise to change was echoed many times in his past. His children came to distrust everything he said and did. Although, he believed that his treatment of his family was for their own good, the family knew it wasn't in their best interest. Even after his wife began to believe that he was actually willing to change, the children remained unconvinced.

The children refused to consider changing their behaviors and attitudes until they felt safe in the knowledge that their father was finally sincere. They confronted him with his past crimes against them one after another. When he listened and accepted his responsibility they began to believe that he might be trusted.

Being his children, they believed that they had the right to punish him for his crimes. It was what he taught them by his actions. They began to escalate, mirroring his violent and unreasonable behavior that they had been the target of throughout their lives.

When they were satisfied that he believed he had been wrong in his treatment of them, they began to change their intent toward the family in general. The belief that the family was worth saving began to grow. Their father demonstrated his change of heart by refusing to retaliate, no matter how outrageously they behaved toward him. He had to admit that they were doing what he taught them. He realized that the only way to teach them another, more loving way was to demonstrate it by his behavior.

At the turning point in the mother's healing process, her intent was to punish her husband because of his insincerity. He convinced her and the children that he was willing to change. They felt betrayed when he didn't. He gave lip service to changing, but his actions stated that he was not willing to take responsibility for himself and his past.

She stubbornly chose death. It was her choice and if it wasn't honored, she felt that she wasn't honored. Her upbringing dictated that she must honor her husband and the only way out of the marriage was death. Her intent was to leave the marriage. Her belief was that the only way out of her suffering was death. She intended to die.

As she prepared for her death, she began to see that she had many reasons to live. She chose to change her belief that she was a failure as a person, mother and wife. With this change of belief came a change in intent. She now intended to live. Her smoking and drinking, however revealed her belief that she may change her mind. She still retained the option to choose death if she had been tricked again, but her intent to heal was greater than her intent to die.

The story above illustrates how aspects of your health - mental, physical, emotional and spiritual may be revealed by being present with what you experience in your body with your own inner senses. It also follows the healing process using the metaphor of family relationships.

The Inner Child

Body sensations provide an easy way to reach your inner child by focusing your awareness on the feelings that occur in your body when you recall a past event. In remembering an event, you experience it and react to it in a way consistent with your beliefs. Inner child work focuses on relationships with yourself as well as with others.

You adopt a physical stance or posturing that affirms your beliefs about the event. If you believe there is danger, your body braces to fight or run away. Your brain signals the rest of your nervous system to speed up certain chemicals and slow others to prepare your body for action.

When you think about an event, your body reacts in a subtle manner as if the original event were happening right now. When you focus on this reaction, the emotional and belief patterns that you originally felt may become clear.

Your physical attitudes, emotions and beliefs reflect how you see yourself, how you feel about yourself and the people in your life, your physical environment, and your spiritual beliefs and practices. Your life challenges are part of the expression of your harmony or lack of harmony with your total environment. You can interact with the physical and emotional expressions of your life challenge the way you might interact with a child - an inner child here.

The purpose is to discover the needs of your inner child, a metaphor for your adult needs, to release the negative emotions or limiting beliefs that are still playing out in your life. Often we were traumatized by something during childhood. Seemingly small events can cause a lasting trauma. A part of our awareness breaks off to protect us from perceived

44

danger. This awareness (a child's awareness) continues to defend itself as long as it believes danger exists. The inner child doesn't realize that he survived and the danger has past. He cannot relax and move on until he feels safe from the danger that may no longer exist. The trauma is preserved in a defensive body posture. The child's defensive posture becomes chronic, low level tension for the adult. The trauma the child defends against may be either actual or imagined but the tension held in body attitude is real and present even if unnoticed. Trauma may also happen to adults from events that seems trivial to others. Trauma may express in a specific part of the body and be held there by beliefs and emotional charges.

One way to think of it is that your inner child is calling out for help in the form of a physical symptom. The longer you ignore the child, the louder he becomes and the more the physical aspect intensifies. The metaphor of the inner child provides a means of releasing chronic stressors that cause adverse health consequences.

Spiritual

There is an aspect of existence that interacts with our bodies and infuses them with life. Without this aspect, our bodies becomes corpses. In practice, this aspect appears to transcend the life of the body in that some people easily experience prenatal states of existence. Others experience what they interpret as past lives. Near death experiences are common.

Kirlian photography reveals some interesting findings about the energetic bodies that appear to infuse everything. When we cut a limb from a plant Kirlian photography shows that from an energy field standpoint, the limb still exists and before a new leaf grows, an energy outline of the mature leaf exists. The material part of the newly forming leaf conforms to and fills the preexisting energy outline. Physical or emotional wounds appear in a person's energy field in a similar way. These wounds often correspond to present life trauma, but sometimes they do not.

Sometimes during closed-eye or altered-states therapy such as hypnosis, people will experience what is commonly thought to be past life trauma as a contributing factor to their current difficulties in life. John, a man with a lifelong explosive temper, found his chronic anger was due to a previous life experience of dying on a battlefield. John felt duped into going to war in the name of God and felt ultimately betrayed as he froze to death in an ice encrusted mud puddle as men rushed by and over him. As he lay there dying, he felt so much anger and hatred toward God that his anger and hatred lasted through a succession of lives as a soldier that lasted for several thousand years. The experience during altered- state therapy helped him release his fear and find a deeper peace which had eluded him all his life.

Gale, a woman with chronic throat problems, experienced being beheaded in ancient Greece. She sensed dying of throat cancer in other lives. Searching her present and past lives, Gale was finding no resolution to her throat problems. When it was suggested that she go to a time and place where she could heal this succession of past life throat conditions Gale experienced what she believed to be a future life where she was healed by a device that emitted sound and light. Gale's throat problem improved after this experience.

Relating to life challenges from the belief in past life trauma allowed healing to happen for these people. Regardless of the validity of reincarnation, working heartfully within whatever system of belief a person presents can bring about profound healing. You can probably think of other possible explanations for these experiences consistent with your beliefs. If past life work provides a way to interact with and heal a life challenge it makes no practical difference if it is literal or metaphoric. Just meet your life challenge, heartfully and without judgment, through any means that presents itself.

Robert O. Becker, M.D., an orthopedic surgeon and medical researcher refers to the current of injury (CI) as a measurable, low voltage, direct current flow of energy that streams from an injury. In an article appearing in the 1991 issue of, *The International Society for the Study of Subtle Energy and Energetic Medicine*, Dr. Becker reported his research into what I call the soft body.

Dr. Becker found a constant field of low voltage, direct current electricity in living beings that interacts with the nervous system. His research supports the idea of an energetic outline existing for an amputated limb that acts as a mold for newly forming tissue. He found that if you cut off a salamander's leg (a salamander can grow a new leg), that an energetic outline of the leg exists with a positive, direct current flow. In a frog (a frog cannot grow a new leg), the same thing happened except the direct current was negative. He also found the more awareness given to the wound, the greater the direct current flow to the injury or energetic outline. He demonstrated this by measuring the CI, or Current of Injury, of the salamander under anesthesia and as it became alert again. Researchers found that reversing the direction of current in the salamander's brain made it unconscious. When they reversed the current flow in an anesthetized salamander, it regained consciousness although the drug was still in the salamander's brain. The degree of consciousness of the salamander was measured by the intensity of the flow of the DC electrical field in its brain. The degree of consciousness or awareness in the wound was measured by the intensity of the flow of electricity in the CI. Thus, the more direct current (awareness) that flowed in the area of the wound, the faster the injury healed.

This highlights the need for pain as part of the healing process. Of course, if the pain is too severe you probably won't listen to it or have any desire to cooperate with it.

Dr. Becker found, in working with people, there are many ways to control the flow of energy in this energetic body, but none worked better in his work than hypnosis. We have the potential to control our energetic bodies by choice. Energy follows awareness. This is a basic of all energy work.

Dr. Becker's research shows the cells, at the end of each nerve ending and neural connection to the spinal cord called Schwann cells, act as communication relays for the soft body. Acupuncture points are usually at these relay stations. Meridians connect these acupuncture points throughout the body. This direct current outline of the soft body may create the energetic outline for the developing physical body. Dr. Becker thinks the direct current field of the energetic body promotes healing. He speculates this energetic body could reach out and touch others and gain knowledge about others through this touch as experienced in the exercises presented here.

To demonstrate, bring any attitude into your awareness. You might choose one that has caused you problems in the past. Perhaps you get angry at your spouse in a certain situation or you feel fearful in different situations. Feel that attitude inside. Notice what happens to your body, your thoughts and your feelings. Allow a person to come to mind. This person will be the appropriate person. It may be someone you met only once thirty years ago, or a celebrity, or anyone else. Notice where on your body this joining is. You may find that the attitude is attached to your heart, or your toes, or any other place, even some that don't seem to be inside your body. It is more important to notice where the attitude attaches to your body than who the original contract was with. If you recognize who is involved in this contract you may choose to release them by name and seal the place of attachment by putting your hand on it and intending that it seal. Each of these connections drain your energy and a color your overall life. Many people may be attached to you in this manner and influence all aspects of your life through these attachments

We can experience how our life energy attaches to various objects, people and ideas. When we infuse an idea with our life energy, it becomes a living being in a way similar to the way our bodies become alive when spirit infuses them. We can attach bits of our life energy to many people, places and ideas. Shamans call this loss of soul and it is used in Shamanistic healing. In our daily lives we infuse many ideas, events, relationships and material objects with our life energy. In the Shaman's view, each bit of attached energy takes away from the energy we have available for living or healing. By attaching some of our energy, we open ourselves to the influence of these outside energies. They become like living beings that survive by consuming our energy and the energy of others who attach to them. Each of these attachments becomes a drain of energy and a source of stress until you release the attachment and withdraw the flow of energy.

As an example, think of someone you've known who was addicted to drama. This is a person who always has a crisis going and wants everyone to join in. Each person who joins in the drama increases the intensity. The intensity can grow and draw more people into the drama. The drama may continue to grow until those who bought into it realize that the event was manufactured and disconnect. The more people that disconnect the smaller the drama becomes.

While you imagine the images offered in the next paragraphs, I invite you to notice the way in which you experience them. Many people, myself included, do not actually see the images as in a dream. Visual images are only one type of imagery. Notice what you do when you pretend or daydream. You may not see an actual image in your mind. It makes no difference what form of imagery you use since you automatically use the form best for you at the moment. The form may change from minute to minute, but you will always find what you need if you are willing to accept it in the form offered. The imagery you use in meditations and in guided imagery will probably match those images you use in daydreaming, planning or remembering.

In the philosophy of Ayurveda all energy has consciousness and all things have energy, so all things have consciousness. Saying that energy follows thought or awareness is a different way of saying that energy is consciousness.

In the spiritual realm all techniques cause changes on all levels. If you intend for something to happen, and you have no opposing beliefs, emotional charges or physical stances, you will cause the thing you intend. Again, the intent brings the awareness of the proper action to cause a goal to become fact in the real world. If you follow the guidance and take this action, you will probably reach your intended goal. If you ignore this guidance and take no effective action, you probably won't reach your goal.

Intent follows awareness which follows intent. Or as the therapeutic touch practitioners say, energy always follows awareness, or energy follows thought, or more simply, energy is awareness. The exercises throughout the book will help you find ways to consciously use your life energy in your daily life.

Dreams

Dreams are an important and readily available means for gaining greater insight into your life challenges. There are many techniques for analyzing dreams, but the most accurate assessment is yours. To understand a particular dream bring yourself to a state of deeper, inner awareness using any method you choose. Move closer and closer to the dream state. When you are ready, bring the dream more into your awareness by making the details sharper and clearer, the sounds more vivid and the feelings more present like turning up the volume, intensity and brightness of your internal monitor.

Begin reviewing the dream from the first part remembered to the last part remembered. Then move from the last part of the dream you remember to the first part. The details become clearer as you progress.

Let your inner wisdom translate the dream as you run it through your awareness again. If some meaning isn't clear, describe each detail of the dream as if talking to a being from outer space who knows nothing of life on earth. How would you describe a dog, a pen or a picnic table to an alien who had no concept of these things? Describe each detail in your dream, no matter how ordinary, as if teaching an alien being. Choose any area of your life and ask yourself how these details fit into what is happening in that part of your life. What do they mean? What action might you take? Ask your higher mind to let this interpretation be about something specific, like your life challenge. If you have questions about the effectiveness of a plan or treatment in dealing with your life challenge, ask that the answer be relevant to the treatment.

Another way to use dreams in your healing is to program your dreaming. One way to do this is to bring your awareness to the life challenge you are working on before you fall asleep at night. Bring as many details into your awareness as you can. Choose to continue the work that you have been doing while you dream. You may, or may not, be aware in your dreams as you direct your immune system and other related aspects of your life. You may find that you understand profound things about your healing and your life energy as you work in this realm on the edge of consciousness. This knowledge, at times, disappears with the first flash of wakefulness. With practice you can recall more vividly the details of your dreams. If you don't recall the work you do in your dreams it doesn't matter. You have still done the work.

Once when I had the flu, a viral strain that most people suffered with for more than a week, I spent about thirty of the next forty-eight hours in a partial lucid dream state. I used sound, light, color and imagery to direct my white blood cells to kill the virus.

Imagery helped me wash the wastes from the dead virus out of my body. I massaged sore muscles with the fingers of my soft body. I applied a healing, soothing salve to my cramped, dehydrated muscles. I used my soft body hands to balance the flow of energy through my body. After the forty-eight hours I was well again.

Had I attended to the warning signs when my body first began to alert me of poor nutrition, I might have avoided the flu. My immune system was weakened. My nutrition was lousy; I was dehydrated from not drinking enough water or providing adequate minerals; I didn't exercise; I wasn't relaxing at home or on weekends. I was aware of my poor lifestyle, but I didn't take heed so my lack of self-respect had to express itself in a more drastic way. If I had continued to ignore these things, I believe that the intent behind the lack of self-respect would have resulted in a louder cry for help from within myself. This cry might have been anything, from a ten-day bout with the flu to pneumonia that would cause me to stop and examine my intent toward my life and myself.

The next time I had the flu many years later I was miserable for 10 days. No matter how hard I worked with these techniques the flu didn't go away until it ran its natural course. This form of healing seldom fails me, but in this case I would have done better to follow the guidance to get a flu shot instead of arrogantly insisting that I didn't need one. My attitude prevented me from me from following valid and wise guidance.

Keeping a journal of drawings, dreams, insights, imagery or thoughts can help you to understand the aspects of different life challenges and how they relate to each other and to the world. Bill, a businessman, saw immediately the reason he sabotaged his efforts in business after he drew a picture of his ideal life. Bill was surprised at what he drew. When he wrote down what he wanted in life, it became clear that the things he had told himself were important weren't really that important to him. Having identified his real intent in life - to enjoy his family first and his business second - made Bill's real intent much easier to fulfill.

The Birth Council

Get comfortable and settle into your body. Begin to move back in time to your childhood moving through time as if it were a river. Float backwards on this river, moving against the current, going back through the different periods of your life. Moving through days, weeks, months and years go back, riding the river of time. Go back to childhood to a time when things were simpler and truth was easier, where there was more potential in the world. Go back to the time when all was potential. Go back through school years, back to the time of being a toddler, to a time when you could barely walk, back to a time of crawling. Go back to infancy, to a time when your muscles were so new that they hardly worked at all. Go back past your birth back into the womb where you were safe and warm in perfect union with your mother. You feel sad because she is sad or feel joyful because she feels joy. Go back, growing smaller and smaller. Listen to the sound of your mother's heart beating becoming dimmer and dimmer until it fades into silence. Go back now to your conception and before. Imagine a birth council of wise beings preparing you for your coming birth. Spend as much time with your council as you choose, asking all the questions that you choose, being open to the knowing of a part of your greater self. Imagery need not be accurate in the objective world to be true and useful in healing.

Take all the time you want and when you're ready allow your eyes to open and your consciousness to return to the room around you.

I Am

This is an adaptation of a traditional Qigong exercise.

I invite you to bring your awareness to your feet. Begin to settle into your body and ground. Let your feeling go deep into the earth. Center yourself in your body. Bring your awareness fully and squarely into your physical body. Quickly take inventory of what's going on inside, starting with your toes and moving upward. No need to do anything. No judgment about anything, just notice what's there. Bring your awareness to the space just in front of your spine and there you'll find a column of light, a string of light that vibrates "I am." Not the little i of your ego, but the big I of your greater self. Bring your awareness into that vibration making it brighter and more intense with each breath, and let the string of light move right down through your pelvic floor and connect with the earth. And let it move out the top of your head and connect with a place in the universe that has the healing energy for you that you need right now.

Tap into that healing place, and let it fill column of light making it grow larger within you. Let it grow larger with each breath, moving outward through your skin, creating a shell of golden light, like an egg around you. Within this shell of golden light you're protected from many things. This shell is always available to you to use any time or place that you choose. Bring the healing energy to the place inside where your life challenge resides. Allow the energy to flow right through your life challenge into the earth, healing you in body, mind and soul as it passes through you. Take as much time as you choose to bathe your life challenge in this healing energy. Observe without needing to do anything, without needing to judge anything or know how it works. Just allow this energy to go through you washing away anything toxic. Wash it away to the core of the earth to be incinerated. Trust your guidance to know what you need to do to heal your life challenge. Take all the time you need or want to work with your life challenge and this healing energy. When you're ready, just allow your eyes to open naturally and easily and return your awareness to the room around you.

Protecting Yourself

Go back into your egg. Notice any holes in your egg where your energy flows outward or where outside energy flows in. Take inventory of all such leaks. You may see them, feel them, or sense them in any other way. You may have feelings or memories associated with these energy leaks. Just notice what you find without the need to do anything about it. You may associate these leaks or flows with other people or situations. The source or nature of the leaks and what or who they are connected with is not important in this exercise. The only thing you need to be concerned with here is sealing the leaks and stopping the energy loss according to your own choice.

When you have located a leak, put your hand on the part of your body where the leak is occurring. Imagine a membrane like a soap bubble. Use your hand to smooth over the hole and seal it so it doesn't leak inward or outward. Continue sealing the holes until all are repaired. You may choose to contemplate the nature of the leaks and how the energy flows through them. It's not important to this exercise. The important thing is to seal the leaks.

If you are aware of no energy leaks, allow your hand to move to a spot on your body. You can trust your hand to go to the right place. Push against your hand with your awareness for a few minutes then repeat.

Loss of Self

An example of loss of self was explained to me by a friend. It was her way of coping in the world. She said, "It's like I have these things I worry about all around me, motioning to her waist to show the worries as being attached to her by strings. When the stress from worrying about one thing becomes overwhelming, I just start worrying about something else. I kind of move around my waist from one set of worries to another." This is loss of self because it drains her life energy.

This is a source of constant and sometimes extreme stress and anxiety in her daily life. She uses most of her energy supporting her circle of worries. The overflowing bags of churning emotion hanging from her waist are carried with her through every daily function weighing her down and sapping her energy. Life for her is tiring and difficult. She invests most of her energy in what she doesn't want and that's what she creates.

I invite you to find a comfortable position and settle into your body. Become aware of whatever supports you, what you're resting on. Feeling gravity, allowing gravity to support you, knowing gravity won't fail you. Relaxing into that knowledge, assurance and trust. Begin to scan your body and take inventory of what's going on right now. Feel all your extremities. Using your inner eye, inner ear and inner touch, check your bone marrow as well as the hard outer layer of your bones. With your inner senses move your awareness at your own speed through your torso and internal organs, all the muscles of your body and all the space inside your body.

Continue to settle into your body and explore. Going through your daily life you expend a certain amount of energy. If you consider all of this energy as a full tank of fuel, notice now where you use your energy. Starting first thing in the morning and proceeding through your day notice where you invest your energy. Notice how much of your fuel is consumed by thinking. Notice the quality of these thoughts. Are they productive thoughts? Are they obsessive thoughts? Do they help you in your daily life? Or do they run you down? Notice if one kind of thought takes more energy than another.

When you perform a task in life, how much energy do you use for thinking, worrying, telling yourself that it's too hard and feeling victimized by having to perform the task? How much of your energy is used in the actual task of doing it. Just notice without judgment or needing to do anything about it. Notice now how much of your energy for the day is invested in other people. How much of your energy do you put into maintaining other people's lives? And how much energy do you put into your possessions? Notice how much of your energy, when you have done all the other things of the day, is left for fulfilling your life, for getting what you want in life. Just notice.

Now bring your awareness to a life challenge. Notice how much of your daily energy is invested in this life challenge. Notice how much of this energy is invested in your relationship with your life challenge. Notice how you feel about it and how you interact with it in your daily life. Notice how much of your energy is consumed by the relationship between your life challenge and the world. Notice how much of the energy that's invested in your life challenge is used for actually healing your life challenge and how much energy is allotted to maintaining it. How much energy is invested in adjusting your life to move toward a healthier you? How much energy do you invest in maintaining the unhealthy aspects of your life? Notice without judgment. Take as much time as you choose to explore and to make changes that you feel are appropriate. When you are ready, just let your eyes open and your consciousness return to the room around you.

Reclaiming Your Energy

Breathe slowly and deeply releasing tension from your body with each exhalation. Infusing your body with strength and vitality with every inhalation. Settle into your body relaxing more with each breath. Become more present and adjust yourself into a truly comfortable position. Feel your breath moving deeper and deeper into your body. Allow your breath to move into your belly, your belly expanding with each inhalation and contracting with each exhalation. Feeling the deliciousness of the sensations as your breath moves through your body. Let your breath move down into your pelvis expanding like the bulb of an eyedropper, expanding at your hips and the front and back of your pelvis and your pelvic floor. Expand with each inhalation. Contract with each exhalation - as if squeezing the bulb of the eyedropper. Let your breath move down through your legs to the bottoms of your feet, then breathe into your arms and hands. Fill your neck and head with breath let your entire skin expand with each inhalation. Contract with each exhalation. Experience your skin as a single unit, flexible and strong, covering your entire body.

You invest your energy in many areas: people, places, things and ideas. These things consume your energy. Bring a person you know into your mind. Notice where on your body where you connect to this person. Maybe you connect from one part of your body or maybe more. Just notice. Bring your awareness to your skin at the place where you connect to this person. Bring more people you know to mind one-by-one and notice where and how you connect with them. Bring places relevant to your life to mind and notice how you connect to these. Bring your possessions to mind and notice from where on your body and how you connect to them. Bring something to mind that you have strong feelings about. Notice how your body connects to these ideas.

Notice which connections serve you and which connections don't. Notice which connections nurture you and which connections drain you. Notice healthy connections and how and where they connect to you. Notice the same about the unhealthy connections. If it's appropriate seal the unhealthy connections so that they can't connect to you again. If it is not appropriate to seal an unhealthy connection make note of why without judgment. Disconnect and seal or strengthen connections following your own guidance to do what's right for you in the present time.

Take all the time you choose to work with these connections, disconnecting and reclaiming your energy and reassigning the way you invest your life energy. Make changes that support healing and being fulfilled as a person, creating the life that you want.

Take all the time you choose to work with these connections. When you're ready allow your eyes to open and your consciousness to return to the room around you.

Community Mind

We infuse our relationships, ideas, beliefs, and material things with our life energy. In a way, we are attached to these things and maintain them as living entities by infusing them with our energy. It's like a complex web of energy exists both inside and outside of our bodies that connects by energetic pathways to other people, ideas, memories and material things to name a few. This is the community mind.

The worldwide web is a small example. People all over the world connect to those people, place, things and ideas that interest them using a dynamic web of energy that can nurture or drain the person who connects. Websites interact almost as living beings whose life is infused into them by the people who connect and feed them with their own energy.

The action of community mind is seen in the insect and animal kingdoms. The efficient team work in ants and bees is well-known. When building a place to live or defending the colony there is only a single mind operating. When a flock of geese fly, they form a V formation to break the wind and conserve energy. There is no set leader of the flock. The lead position is constantly being filled by a different bird. The whole flock operates as a single mind. Schools of fish do the same.

As humans we are connected by the common mind of our family, peers and society. By shared beliefs, the community mind sets the limits or boundaries of acceptable behavior and experience. In any given setting, we can usually tell how acceptable we are without having to ask anyone. We tend to unconsciously adjust our beliefs about ourselves and the outside world so we fit in. This can cause contradictory beliefs that may result in chronic stress that can affect a person's health. The opposite is also true. If societal, family, or peer group beliefs are in harmony with our self-image a feeling of well-being can result, even if we must ignore incongruences with perceivable reality.

Most people in our society share a belief in chairs. If you place a chair in a room and bring in a thousand people to view the chair, each person sees a chair. Some see a comfortable chair, others see an antique chair, and some see a wooden chair and so on. Each view is personal and different but somehow congruent.

Emotional

Emotions are powerful forces in our lives. They can overcome the best reasoning and understanding of any situation and leave us looking foolish. The wiring for emotions exists in our brains long before the circuitry for intellect develops. All circuitry for speech and visual processing pass through the emotional part of the brain. The neural impulses passing through these circuits are subject to emotional clearance and censoring before they go to the thinking area of the brain. The emotional part of the brain may control the circuitry to all but basic life support functions by blocking the passage of neural impulses. Everyone has experienced impaired judgment from anger, fear, guilt or jealousy. Your immune system, in essence, feels the same emotions as the larger you feels. Any emotional impairment also impairs your immune system. Bringing emotion into awareness, with the intent of changing in a healthier way, promotes healing and the awareness of the actions needed for further healing. Like the sensations of your physical body, your emotions are an accurate map to your overall state of being.

Emotions play your body like a musical instrument and create kinesthetic images within your body. As you focus on your emotions in a given situation, the ways in which they reach into the different facets of your life will begin to become more apparent. Some people refer to this web of emotion that resonates within as the emotional body. The beliefs and choices associated with your emotions become clearer as you become more aware of your emotional body.

Bring a strong emotion to mind and notice how it fits into your body. A study where people were asked to color the location and intensity of emotions in their bodies on a paper template revealed that we all experience emotions in the same parts and intensities in our bodies.

Another way of looking at the emotional body is from transpersonal psychology. Stanislov Grof, M.D., assigns all experiences to COEXs or compressed systems of experience. Each COEX contains sensory, biographical, perinatal and transpersonal experiences that are related and have a common emotional charge that they organize around. These systems of experience are held together by a common emotional charge. Emotional charges that adversely affect health may be accessed through the various aspects of the COEX including sensory components, the verbal story we tell ourselves about it and any associated trauma. The story of any aspect of the emotional body can be told in many ways that are both verbal and non-verbal. Releasing the common emotional charge releases the COEX as an energetic event. The charge may be released by changing the supporting verbal beliefs or by adjusting non-verbal aspects.

Beliefs and Emotions

Beliefs and emotions are presented together, because in real life they are inseparable. When working with the physical body, beliefs and emotions may emerge.

You can examine beliefs and change those beliefs that do not serve you. Maybe they served you at one time or maybe they resulted from mistaken assumptions. It doesn't matter. You can change your beliefs by choice as long as the new beliefs doesn't violate your general belief system. For example, if you have a belief that you live in the best city in the world, it follows that your sports team must be the best, regardless of winning or losing. If you move to a different city you may adjust your beliefs making your new team the best, because you live in the best city in the world, regardless of what city that is. Your feelings change with your beliefs.

Milton Erickson, MD used a process he called reframing, or changing the meaning of an event, to adjust beliefs. There are two forms of reframing: content and context. One example of context and content reframing comes from Erickson's work with a young girl with a wart on her hand. The wart had resisted all treatment. He found that the girl's grandfather, who had recently died, had accidentally brushed the back of her hand with his cigar on the spot where the wart formed. Erickson told the girl that the wart was a gift from her grandfather. This is content reframing: changing the wart from a large problem involving dragging the child to doctors to a gift or something to cherish. The meaning of the wart changed. Erickson also told the girl she should keep this precious gift until she finished grieving for her grandfather. It was her grandfather's way of staying with her a little longer. Erickson explained that her grandfather wanted her to let go of him gradually now that he was gone. The wart disappeared after several weeks. This example of context reframing, or redefining, changed the child's relationship with the wart.

Beliefs that limit or restrict a person can restrict deep healing. A single limiting belief can hold a person hostage. One belief can prevent healthy change or cause a person to behave in ways that are harmful. Sometimes beliefs naturally fade away as we grow and learn more to be replaced by updated beliefs. A person may also cling to a belief against overwhelming evidence. We can choose to adjust or release limiting beliefs as we discover them. We can also choose to keep them.

It can be revealing to state what you believe about your life challenge. The results are usually surprising. Take a pencil and paper and begin to write about your life challenge. Write quickly without worrying about style, grammar or making sense. Write for twenty minutes without stopping. Just write whatever comes into your mind. You are free to throw this paper away without showing it to anyone. Write for another fifteen minutes from the point of view of your life challenge.

When you are in touch with a life challenge, you can usually state the beliefs associated with it. Common beliefs that might surface are, I am no good; I deserve punishment; I am not lovable; I am not worthy; I don't belong or I am not welcome. You can recognize these and other limiting beliefs in your life if you listen for them. Notice that each of these phrases causes an emotional response when you say them to yourself. Repeat them several times and notice the way your posture and feelings change as you read each. Sometimes you can change beliefs by simply stating them and choosing to change them.

You can access beliefs through emotions. Bring your feelings about any subject to mind. If you find fear there is a supporting belief that there is danger. Notice what the danger is. Is the danger real? What makes you feel that there is danger? You may be able to follow the chain of beliefs to their origin.

You can also access emotions through beliefs. Bring any aspect of your life to mind and notice what you believe about it. For example, if you bring a time that someone betrayed you to mind and notice what you believe about the situation you may find a belief is that you deserved to be betrayed. You may have beliefs supporting feelings of unworthiness or unlovability. Feeling the emotions invokes the beliefs that trigger the emotions.

Anatomy of Anger

Anger is our natural reaction to fear that drives us to overcome its paralyzing effects so we can face the danger that it represents. In some instances anger is a sane and healthy emotion, but chronic anger can contribute to many diseases and daily maladies.

When the world we experience doesn't match the world as we believe it is stress results. Our realities tend to conform to our beliefs regardless of any evidence to the contrary. When the reality outside ourselves is in conflict with our beliefs stress hormones, cortisol and norepinephrine, are released. These are useful fight or flight drugs, but chronic elevated levels in your system can contribute to heart disease, cancer, diabetes and other mental and physical health problems. Chronic stress can also contribute to unhealthy expression of DNA. When the world outside doesn't match our beliefs the healthiest response is to acknowledge the discrepancy and adjust our beliefs accordingly.

Our nature is to stick with our beliefs despite our objective experience. We choose our beliefs for our own reasons. As infants and children we choose beliefs because they are modeled by those older than us. Our survival depends on accepting the reality of our elders when we are small. Adjusting our beliefs to match objective reality can threaten the basic foundations of our realities.

As we grow older we begin to choose beliefs that differ from our family's realities as we have experiences outside of our family's influence. Chronic stress from dissension between family members may result as the hypocrisy of family beliefs compared to real life experience is uncovered. We people are not good at admitting our own hypocrisy. That requires facing the fact that everything we believe may not be true. The stress from chronic discrepancy between objective reality and the reality defined by our beliefs will evolve into fear if not resolved. We choose our beliefs for our own reasons. The fact that a belief contradicts our perceivable reality may, or may not, be sufficient reason to alter the belief.

If we don't resolve the stress of contradictory realities fear results. Something is threatening. In this case it is the inconsistency between our beliefs and objective reality that threatens our worlds. If the source of the fear is not resolved it will turn into anger to spur us into action to escape the danger and resolve the fear.

A lifetime of unresolved anger will likely lead to an early and painful death. Anger may be useful when there is action to be taken to escape danger. When the danger is facing the hypocrisy of our contradictory beliefs, it becomes much more complicated than killing it or running from it. The tricky thing about hypocrisy is that it's so easy to see in others and so difficult to see our own.

If we manage to resolve the contradiction of our beliefs the anger disappears. The danger no longer exits. It may have only existed as a byproduct of conflicting ideas made real by imagination. When we believe the danger no longer exists our fear subsides. If there is no fear, there is no anger.

New fear may result from the realization that you have lived your life based on beliefs that you now alter or release. You may be angry with those who helped form the beliefs that you have come to doubt. You can choose to take responsibility and move on or you can choose to be a victim whose life has been thwarted by those who misled you perpetuating your fear.

Our beliefs are like protecting spheres whose boundaries border on all sides of our total knowledge, containing all that we know or are capable of knowing. Beyond that is our ignorance, what we don't know and what we are incapable of knowing. Outside the boundaries of our beliefs we find the fear of the unknown, the unknowable and the uncontrollable. Whenever we grow as individual's we experience fear. Acknowledging your fear and moving through it prevents getting stuck in it.

The Boundaries of Belief; The Prison of Emotion

Our beliefs determine how we experience our realities. It's as if the scenery we pass through in our life's journey is painted on the canvas of our minds and projected around us. The mechanics of vision show how this works. When we open our eyes and see the world, what our eyes are seeing and what our mind's eye is seeing are two different things. Our physical eyes pick up images that are upside down and distorted. The images from our eyes are transmitted to our brains where they are turned right side up and stretched out. Our brains fill in the details in a way that conforms to what we believe. We choose what we overlook by what we pay attention to. We fit any experience into our belief systems regardless of if the experience is in fact consistent with what we believe. We will make it consistent. We are masters of fitting the square peg into the round hole.

All experiences are somehow contained within the boundaries of our beliefs. We choose how we feel about what we find within our belief boundaries. Our bodies react in ways that are consistent with our beliefs. Of course every person sees, feels and reacts in their own unique way. Every event we experience fits into our belief systems, as well as, everyone else's belief systems no matter how contradictory their experiences are to ours. We experience according to what we believe.

We selectively tune out much of our daily world. The only way we can describe anything to ourselves is with the words and ideas we know. We overlook anything that doesn't fit our beliefs because to us it doesn't exist. If we are aware enough to notice something contradictory, we must alter it to fit our beliefs. If we can't describe it to ourselves we can't fix it into our minds nor make memories of it. In some ways if we can't put words to it, we can't make it exist.

A recent study suggests that children in affluent households have a vocabulary of 20,000 words by the time they are 6-years-old while children from poor households have a vocabulary of only 5,000 words. This gives the children from affluent households 15,000 more concepts and nuances, 15,000 more tools in life. These children's worlds are much larger than those of the ghetto child. This gives them 15,000 ways that the boundaries of their worlds are bigger, but the outer boundaries of their worlds are still limited by their beliefs and the concepts they support.

There is a movie entitled, *The Gods Must Be Crazy*. The story is about an empty Coke bottle that was discarded from an airplane somewhere above a remote village in Africa. The people of the village knew nothing about glass or soft drink bottles. When they found the bottle, they viewed it as a gift from the gods that rode in the great shiny, noisy birds. In their belief system there were no referent ideas for airplanes or bottles. The nearest this foreign object came to fitting into their belief system and language was as a gift from the gods.

People in the village began to treasure the bottle. New emotions such as jealousy and violence erupted. After months of turmoil, they finally sent a man to throw it off the edge of the world and return it to the gods. The bottle fit into their belief system in ways that were harmful to the villagers. The new emotions were dangerous and they chose to remove the source of the problem. Another choice would have been to change the meaning of the bottle so it had little or no emotional charge.

Ingrained in each belief is an emotional charge. When we have conversations, the beliefs associated with the words we use evoke in us the emotional charges and physical attitudes we attribute to the words. If we use angry words we feel angry and defiant. We may clench our fists, plant our feet firmly and tighten our jaws and stomach muscles. If we are recalling a difficult situation, our bodies and emotions may react as if it was happening right now. Along with an emotional charge, each belief expresses itself with facial expressions, physical attitudes and stress or wellbeing neurochemicals. We always have the option of adjusting our attitude associated with any situation thereby adjusting the supporting belief along with its meaning and emotional associations.

Our bodies reflect our emotions. If we find ourselves in difficulty or danger, we tense and brace to flee or to do battle. Our stress hormone levels rise. Our hearts race and our breathing rates increase. We become highly alert and energized. If we feel safe and comfortable, the opposite occurs.

After birth, we accept the beliefs of our parents and siblings as a matter of survival. Of course, we can't question these beliefs. We don't possess the verbal skills to question anything. We use these early nonverbal, emotional beliefs as the basic framework for our later beliefs. As infants, we fill this framework with verbal belief as best we can as our word skills develop. We may figure out that the sun sleeps when we do so if we don't sleep the sun won't come out. We may adopt this belief and hold it against all logic because it makes our world of beliefs consistent.

The way we often experience the world is like going to Hawaii, staying in a hotel room, reading about the marvels that exist outside the door but not having the time to experience them because we are too busy narrating descriptions of the wonders outside even though we've never seen them.

We have all experienced discovering that we believed something was ridiculous, but with our level of reasoning skill it was the closest we could come to understanding at the time. This understanding somehow fit into our framework of belief. Santa Claus is a good example. When we discover contradictory beliefs the healthy response is to adjust our beliefs to be more functional.

All beliefs rely on supporting beliefs. No single belief stands alone. Each belief exists in its own environment and is altered by any change in supporting beliefs. Before you can believe that you can run you must believe that you can stand and walk. You must also believe that running is possible. If you injure a knee and believe that you can no longer walk without a cane, you don't believe you can still run and you may never try running again. Every belief about your ability to move your body is altered by the belief you can walk only with a cane. Until you prove to yourself that you can run again, you are burdened with a limited belief about running.

If you notice, you will probably find that you go through life describing every detail to yourself. You may describe the most common things to yourself as if you had never seen them before. You experience the world directly; you are aware of what you experience, but you are still compelled to describe what you have experienced over and over again buffering yourself from directly experiencing the world.

We choose our beliefs for our own reason that often have nothing to do with objective reality. We may choose beliefs for reasons as frivolous as they make people laugh. Mostly we choose beliefs that allow us to fit in with those around us. We may just accept the group beliefs without much thought to their validity. A basic precept of psychology is that people do things for their own reason. That includes choosing and adjusting beliefs.

Intellectual

The intellectual realm is your belief system. Your beliefs are your internal images of your world as you have come to expect it to behave. You have many beliefs which you aren't aware of, but these beliefs still operate in your life. Your beliefs determine the way you relate to the world - self-talk, body posture, emotional stance, musculature, attitude, quality of movement, etc. These aspects reflect your beliefs about reality.

You change your beliefs through awareness. When you bring a belief into awareness, you may update the belief according to your current understanding and intent in life. You release a belief when there is no remaining belief structure to support it. At times, entire limiting belief structures collapse by releasing a single supporting belief. When you learned there was no Santa Claus that single change caused the collapse of an entire set of beliefs. If there was no Santa, then there was no Rudolph, no Mrs. Claus, and no elves and so on. Maybe that brought the suspicion that there were other lies you believed and were part of your basic foundation in life.

It can be terrifying knowing that your sense of yourself and the outside world are based on lies. We seem to have a safety feature that allows us to collapse outdated belief systems at a rate that prevents psychosis. Children seldom go into a deep depression when they realize their parents lied to them about Santa and the Easter Bunny. They may mourn the loss, but the betrayal will probably be buried in their minds.

The betrayal may return later in another form like a seemingly irrational anger or distrust of adults. As you get older, you may gradually release the belief that you can't trust adults, but you may find that you still don't trust certain people like teachers, principals, doctors, judges, preachers, police or others in positions of authority. This can be source of chronic low level stress that can harm your health.

We embrace and release beliefs only according to our choice or intent to do so. We maintain beliefs by choice. Stress occurs when we hold opposing beliefs to those of our families, societies or ourselves. This may express as mental or physical health problem. Being against yourself is a hard position to maintain.

The Secret

The secret is a powerful force. You adjust your life to protect your secrets. Even if it's that little savings fund you've hidden from your spouse, a secret causes stress in your life. If your secret is that your parents are raging alcoholics and you are under constant threat of someone finding out, the stress increases. James Pennebaker, Ph.D., Professor of Psychology at Southern Methodist University, says suspects often thank lie detector operators for helping them to confess. They experience a profound relief when they no longer have to bear their deepest criminal secrets.

Family secrets can be deadly. A woman who had undergone a double mastectomy was told by her doctors she had only a short time to live. She made it clear that this cancer was not about her, it was about her family. The way they treated each other was killing her and she would die if the family battles didn't stop. She stated her conditions for living, "I am going to die if these guys don't start learning how to get along. They don't have to be perfect. They just have to try to really care." As the family confessed their secrets they began to communicate about previously taboo subjects she began to change. Honest talk started between family members. As her family moved toward better health, she also became less stressed and healthier. The cancer went into remission. Although her family was still having problems, they were making progress.

Self-Talk

The power of internal dialogue is well-known. Within our realities nothing that exists is without a supporting belief. Thus, we experience only that which we believe. If we have no belief that allows something exists, we will not perceive it. A belief is a part of the template that we use to experience our worlds. All experience is compared to our personal templates and what can't be forced to fit is discarded. Everyone experiences an event differently as you'd expect when all observers fit the experience into their own unique belief system. At crime scenes, police often get a different story and description of the suspects from each witness. Each witness adapts the experience to fit into his own belief system. What he sees is a second-hand explanation of what happened consistent with his beliefs and self-talk. Even though he witnessed the event first-hand, his belief takes precedence over his sensory experience. It's possible to experience first-hand without the filters of belief, but we rarely do that. It's confusing and stressful when we notice the gaps between our beliefs and the objective world often resulting in falling asleep and forgetting the event as if it were a dream. Being present to act in the world instead of reacting to our self-talk allows us to escape the blinders of our beliefs.

Our words become the boundaries of our beliefs and therefore our experience. For example, if our self-talk revolves around being a victim without control over our lives, we are anxious and feel lost. We draw victimizers into our lives or create them by explaining to ourselves how others take advantage of us. We know other choices exist, but we selectively experience life within the boundaries of our own belief systems. If we live within a victim bubble, the beliefs available within this framework will make us victims.

As victims, we see only the filled parking spaces and not the empty ones. If we do see the empty spaces, we may whine to ourselves that if we park in these spaces, someone may break into our car or steal it. If we believe that people will take advantage of us, we may exclude people from our lives who care about us and treat us with respect. Caring people don't fit into our view of the world so we settle for those who abuse us. We imprison ourselves within the boundaries of the beliefs we choose.

Our beliefs support and define our emotions and attitudes. When we act within the confinement of our belief systems, we are unable to be present in the moment. We trap ourselves in thinking about the past or rehearsing the future draining our energy with ideas that take us away from here and now. We react in the moment according to our beliefs, attitudes and emotional charges leaving us blind to the here and now present reality. In this way we limit ourselves.

Affirmations

A popular technique to counter negative beliefs is to use positive affirmations. For example, we may say, "I never get what I want," which we may counter with, "I always get what I want." This simply creates another boundary and limits our awareness and options in the world. Always getting what we want is as limiting and maybe more potentially dangerous to us than never getting what we want. Our conscious minds can be as immature as a child's mind. Imagine what would happen if we got every childish, selfish or insensitive wish, or the stress from the world not cooperating by giving us everything we want.

Positive affirmations may be a step toward healing, but the next step is to learn to escape the confines of our beliefs, emotions and attitudes. This is easier than overpowering negativity with positivity. When you have a thought that doesn't serve you, you can make up an affirmation. You might say, "I see the good in all people," and repeat this to yourself until you have overwhelmed the original thought. Or you can simply say something like, "I choose to release that thought, belief, attitude or feeling and its roots." As people we tune into the thoughts of those around us and we may pick up on the negative thoughts of others. We can choose to let any thought or emotion pass us by. No matter where the thought originated we can choose to accept it, or not accept it, as our own.

Affirmations are a shifting of the boundaries of experience and possible action in life. Releasing boundaries also releases limitations. As you choose to release thoughts, emotions, attitudes and beliefs, you may feel like something is leaving your body. This release is an energetic and electrochemical event. When you choose to release that which you have embraced on a superficial level in your life, it may feel like something is floating away from you. If you choose to release something leftover from childhood, it may feel as if something profound has been released from the depths of your body. You may shudder as you feel it migrating through your entire body on its way out. A feeling of relief and having a weight lifted may pervade your being. The experience is different for each person in each situation.

You may also find it helpful to withdraw your life energy from whatever you have released and to seal the energetic pathway of this connection to shield yourself from reconnection. It helps to put your hand on the spot on your body where you connect to the belief, situation, person, place or thing. Press against your hand with your awareness and choose to seal the energy drain.

As you release beliefs and attitudes you become quieter inside. Your awareness of yourself and the outside world becomes increasingly clear. As you become more sensitive to the experiences in your life, more resources become available to you. More choices become available, and it's easier to act in the world with presence. The more you take notice of these subtle sensory sensations, the more you make choices from the reality of here and now instead of the illusions of past and future. Your thoughts and actions become less limited by beliefs and emotions.

Whenever you release something, it's very important to replace it with something you want or want more of in your life. As Wind Woman says, "Nature loves a vacuum. It will rush to fill it - if you empty your basket and don't refill it with what you choose, it will fill with even more of the same poobah you just emptied."

When you release a rude thought you may say, I choose to replace this with self-respect. If you release an angry, unreasonable attitude, you may choose to replace it with a peaceful reasonable attitude. Some useful replacements are: presence, health, patience, kindness, compassion, strength, prosperity, fun, love, humor, knowledge or anything else you find appealing.

Affirmations can be powerful expressions of intent. Use affirmations to clarify that which you choose to move toward as opposed to creating limiting beliefs of what you don't want. I choose to have more fun in my life, is an effective affirmation. I choose to not be so unfun, is not.

When you release something and choose something else to replace it, you are automatically using affirmations. Key words are single words or phrases that bring into awareness the various sensory images of your intent. For example, if you are working on healing, you may choose the word healthy to bring into your awareness your complete sensory image of what being healthy means to you. It's most desirable to clearly express your intent on a preverbal level to avoid the limitations of language. The words you use to describe something flavor it with the beliefs that those words represent to you. Words, with their many nuances, can also spike it with unwanted energy. Expressing your intent in nonverbal forms like: images, feelings, sounds or motion bypasses the constraint of words.

We commonly associate consciousness or awareness with thought. It's as if we believe that if we cease thinking, we will cease to exist. Sub vocal thinking is a necessary expression of consciousness, but there are many other expressions of consciousness such as feeling, emoting, seeing, visualizing, imagining and artful expression. All life is an expression of consciousness. Native Americans believe that all things have consciousness. This must be true if the religions that believe in the oneness of all things, that all is of God, are right. The real power of the techniques presented in this book have nothing to do with thought, they all have to do with awareness. As you read the exercises and ideas, allow yourself to experience them with all your senses. To rely on thinking is an inefficient way of operating in the world. When you use your nonverbal senses, you are more efficient at most things. There are, of course, times when verbal thought is the best tool, such as when doing statistics or preparing a meal from a recipe. One way to view thinking is as a computer program that translates each step and command into people language. Working nonverbally is like using the machine language that has no need for the extra step of translating everything into people language to operate. When performing a task with a computer, the machine language or hardware programming is much faster and more efficient than a computer coding language that uses English to control functions. We learn how to operate the hardware of our body long before we learn to talk. We have the capacity of functioning nonverbally much of the time and yet we choose to mainly limit ourselves to a verbal world.

For example, it's more powerful to see yourself in a new job where you can hear the sounds, see and smell the surroundings, than to tell yourself over and over, I want a new job. When you imagine the new job with all the sensory detail you can muster, you are more likely to recognize and take the action needed to get the job instead of just repeating the affirmation. Of course, if you don't act you won't get the job regardless of whatever else you do. If you take action to get what you want in the world yet tell yourself that you can't possibly succeed, or someone will take it away from you, it is much harder to effectively act. Constant self-defeating chatter drains energy and vitality.

Changes you tell yourself are made for the benefit of others only serve to create more limits in your life. When you give to, or serve others, you are doing it for yourself because who you are demands that you offer service to express yourself in the world. To the person receiving your gift, it feels as though you are doing something kind for them. If you believe you are doing this good deed for someone else and you deserve something in return, you have changed it from a gift to a one-sided contract. It's like saying, I have done this for the universe and I deserve this much in return. It's a fool's contract, like painting a house at random and demanding the owner pay for the work. This attitude puts you in the position of being a victim. When you understand that the reward of serving is in the act of serving not in return payment, you are in a position of partnership and support with the universe.

Belief

When working with any life challenge it may be helpful to discover your beliefs about it. The beliefs you choose set the limits of what you can know about your life challenge. They also limit the action you can take in response to your life challenge. The beliefs you hold are like theatrical scenery that you superimposed on the world around you. You act in your personal drama according to these beliefs. If you believe it is impossible to change your life to a more healthful way, you won't find the guidance nor the resources necessary to adjust your life in a healthier way. It isn't that these resources don't exist. Your lack of supporting belief simply leaves you blind to them. When the oncologist says that your cancer isn't serious and is treatable, you hear the doctor saying, "You have cancer and you're going to die and there isn't any hope for you." The belief (thinking) and emotion associated with the cancer have to be passed through before reason and good judgment are possible. When you are stuck at the belief and emotional level the fear, anger and stress may overwhelm clear thinking.

It's like being given a calculus problem and you only have basic arithmetic to work with. Still, you keep on trying to find the solution. Similarly, in daily life, you may invest your energy in endless thinking - If I were any good I'd be more successful, but if I were successful I would make a lot of money and people with money are bad so I can't be successful, but if I were any good I'd be successful. Your beliefs take away the chance of getting what you want in life. Changing any one of these beliefs expands your world and provides more potential. Money is only one measure of success in life. Many people do very good things in the world with their money. Adjusting supporting beliefs to any one of these can provide more satisfying outcomes.

An example of limiting beliefs is the circus elephant. A thin rope tied to one of its legs holds the immature elephant. As a baby, the elephant is incapable of breaking the rope or pulling the stake from the ground.

As the elephant grows, it believes that the rope is unbreakable though it has enough strength to snap the rope with a single tug. An old belief holds the elephant captive overwhelming present reality.

We tend to hold ourselves captive by beliefs that have no basis in any reality other than our own choice to believe them. Yet, we can update our beliefs and release the damaging attitudes and emotional charges by simply examining the beliefs in light of new knowledge. We can also do tasks that we believe are impossible if we are unaware that we are doing them.

A Russian weight lifter broke a world record after his trainer told him the weight on the bar was lower than the record weight. He had lifted this lower weight many times before. He easily lifted the world record weight though he had never lifted as much before and believed that it was not possible for him to do so.

Throughout history each generation does feats thought impossible by the previous generations. When beliefs change enough to allow the impossible to become the possible, the actual feat often follows closely. Extreme sports are an example. Fifty years ago no one in their right mind would have thought of doing aerial acrobatics on bicycles, motorcycles, skis, skateboards etc. Each generation of extreme athlete does things the last generation never dreamed of. The impossible becomes the ordinary.

Every mind/body exercise you do reveals certain aspects of your beliefs. If you see in your mind's eye that your life challenge is a bear and you are a wounded lamb the belief that you are powerless in the face of your life challenge is apparent. You will be powerless to affect your life challenge in a healthful way until you redefine the relationship between it and you.

A simple exercise for discovering your beliefs about your health and healing is to make a list of your thoughts about a life challenge. The beliefs that emerge may be surprising. Each belief about your life challenge holds an innate intent and imposed limitations to healing. Listing your beliefs on paper or verbally is revealing. State each belief as, "I believe___" Some suggestions are:

- I believe my life challenge serves me by -
- I believe my life challenge hinders me by -
- I believe my life challenge teaches me -
- I believe others see my life challenge as -

• I believe this is how I feel about my life challenge -
• I believe this is what my life challenge means about me -
• I believe my life challenge interferes with what I want in life by -
• I believe that to live to be 100 -
• I believe my family and friends think this about my life challenge -
• I believe people treat me differently because of my life challenge by –
• I believe the motto that my family lives by is –
• I believe the motto that I live by is -
• I believe if my life could be any way that I choose -
• I believe I intend to achieve this in my life -
• I believe pain makes me -
• I believe pain does this to my life -
• I believe my life challenge gives me permission to do or say these things that I wouldn't do or say without it –

Verbal Probes

Verbal probes are an effective way to discover beliefs about your life challenge. Probes are phrases that are supportive and positive. A probe is an offering of emotional nourishment. You react to the probe according to your beliefs and emotional charges about the related issue.

A sample probe might be something like, "You are perfect the way you are." The reaction could be anything from a sigh of contentment to an outburst of anger and tears. Notice how you feel about these words as they apply to you.

To deliver a probe, ask yourself (or the receiving person if you are working with another person) to go inside and become a silent reporter. A reporter does not make judgments or interfere in any way, he just records all that he observes. Ask yourself or the other person to notice any reactions to the probe. Some reactions may include words, images, feelings, realizations, or the relaxing or tensing of muscles. Close your eyes. When you are (your partner is) ready, slowly say the probe, pause a moment then offer the probe again. Notice the reactions without judging them as you hear the words.

Some probes you might find useful are:
•I am (you are) perfect just the way I am
•I am (you are) (lovable, acceptable, worthy)

•I don't need to change to be (lovable, acceptable, worthy)

•I may (you may) claim a treasure from my (your) relationship with my (your) life challenge

•It is okay to heal now

•It is okay not to heal until I am (you are) ready

•It is okay to keep my (your) life challenge until I (you) no longer need it

All probes should be supportive and free of judgment. *Body-Centered Psychotherapy, The Hakomi Method,* by Ron Kurtz has a more complete list of probes and information on the use of probes.

Draw Your Beliefs

Drawing your life challenge can reveal unconscious beliefs. You don't need to be an artist. The crudest picture will do just fine. Draw pictures of:

•Yourself

•Your life challenge

•The action you have taken to heal

•Your immune functions as they interact with your life challenge.

Draw a second set of pictures of the people in your life and how they support you in your healing process. Use crayons of as many colors as you want. Using crayons helps bypass your logical, thinking mind.

These drawings can reveal many beliefs, attitudes and emotional charges. Notice the color or lack of color in the drawing. If color is sparse, this may show a lack of enthusiasm in life. If the picture is full of color, this may suggest an excitement about life and a desire to live. Red may show emotion or conflict. Black may be grief or depression. White on white paper may represent a cover-up or denial or feeling invisible. Yellow might be energy. Orange can suggest change. Purple may show spirituality or support. Blue, green and brown may be neutral. These representations are only guidelines. Consider the colors available as they may be inaccurate in specific drawings. If the only color available is black, it would be ridiculous to consider it a sign of depression. Different colors mean different things in different cultures. What do the colors mean to you? How do they feel to you?

The body of the pictured person may give clues to a problem. If a person in the drawing lacks eyes, he may be hiding something or hiding from something. If the drawing has no feet, this might show a feeling of being stuck or unable to move. The lack of hands may show a feeling of being powerless. A missing nose may show inability to take in nourishment or life force. Missing ears might represent an unwillingness to listen or learn. Drawing only a part of the body where there is ample paper for a full body, may show a feeling of something missing or the inability to take an active part in the healing process. What is missing in the drawing can as important as what is drawn.

If your life challenge is shown in a form that is more powerful than you or the treatment, it suggests that your life challenge is in control. If the drawing shows the immune functions as stronger than the life challenge, control over the life challenge is suggested.

The drawing of the support system may reveal the outside resources available to the person. The barriers caused by beliefs about the intent of the social environment and emotional charges associated with other people and relationships may be revealed. If your drawings show negative aspects, redraw the picture to change them.

Physical

Your body entails the most solid aspects of your being. However, your body isn't solid. Even your bones, if viewed in time lapse, are in a constant state of flux. According to modern physics, the empty space in the human body, at an atomic level, is in proportion to the empty space in the universe. Your body is the slowest vibrating manifestation of your total being. It's the physical expression of all the aspects of your beliefs and the innate expression of your unique humanness.

Your body is the most concrete part of your greater self and may provide clues about the greater you. It is the most available and accurate guide to the action necessary for any healing. Your body is also the place where toxins deposit and where physical repairs take place. Physical movement enhances most healing. Cleaning diseased and distressed tissue and making repairs to your body requires blood flow. Increased blood flow usually boosts healing. All activities in your body rely on oxygen. Increasing air flow through your lungs increases oxygen in your blood and to your individual cells.

Appropriate exercise is helpful in healing any life challenge. You can exercise your body mentally or physically. Your brain acts the same doing either. Professional athletes imagine performing tasks to learn to do them more quickly and proficiently. A golfer may see the entire course in his mind before the tournament imagining each shot. A skier will see and feel each turn in a course in her mind before leaving the starting gate. People who imagine doing exercise, or even intently watch someone else doing exercise, get most of the benefit of the exercise.

It's more common to hear someone say. "I hate exercise.", than it is to hear, "I love exercise." You can exercise like an adult and make it drudgery or you can play like a child and get the benefits of both play and exercise. Make exercise in your mind and body fun. Add humor. Approach it as a child just learning to use her body.

Working with the Physical Body

Your physical body is a quick and accurate guide to your emotions and beliefs. Your body carries memories of the trauma, physical and mental, that it has experienced in the past. A person physically assaulted as a child will usually turn their face quickly away from an approaching hand even if the hand is moving very slowly and the person's eyes are closed. Any physical wounds may have disappeared, yet the wound still exists as an emotional charge in the body triggering an automatic flight reaction.

A person's beliefs reflect in body posture and attitude. A defiant person pushes his chin forward restricting his breathing. To check this out, take a deep breath and notice how deeply you inhale. Now, push your chin forward one inch and notice what happens to your breathing. This chronic breathing pattern, by itself, has long-term health consequences. When you add restricted blood flow from tight shoulder and neck muscles and the frequent anger-kicks of adrenaline and stress neurotransmitters into the bloodstream, it's easy to see how prolonged defiance is harmful to your health.

Beliefs that produce fear and the resulting anger probably produce poor eating habits and abuse of substances such as food, alcohol, tobacco, caffeine and other drugs. Your attitudes directly affect your health. The physical aspects of attitude and belief may be discovered by bringing your awareness to your physical body and using it to guide you toward healing.

Settle into your body and connect with something solid like the floor or the earth. Bring your awareness into your body and release all thoughts of past or future events. Bring your awareness into the present. Probe your body with your awareness and locate a place of pain, tension or distress. Bring your awareness to it with the intent that it heal. Release any emotion or belief related to the pain. Bathing the pain in your awareness and intent to heal is the most direct and powerful technique. Most people need to translate the pain and intent into symbols that provide more concrete tools to work with. Words, visual images, feelings, sounds, movement patterns and colors are sensory symbols that may be used to discover the story of the life challenge and express intent for it to heal.

Squeaky Wheel

To begin any mind/body healing it is helpful to become more aware of your mind/body. I invite you to settle into your body and notice what's going on. Our bodies have a wonderful guidance system that allows us to feel and otherwise sense and experience the signals that something is not right. You can trust yourself to present current, potential, and developing problems in the order of most in need of attention first. The old adage, the squeaky wheel gets the grease, applies.

Settle deeper into your body and listen and feel for the squeaky wheel. You may find pain, tension, irritation, tickling or other things. Whatever you find is right. Let it be whatever it is without judgment. Bring your awareness to the aspect you find in your body that is the most intense, or most painful, or loudest, the part of your body that is the most demanding of your attention.

There is nothing to do about what you find right now. Just experience whatever you find. Go to the first area that calls you. Notice what you feel and what you sense with inner eye and inner ear. Spend as much time as you choose moving from the loudest area, to the next loudest, to the next. Maybe you will follow the next squeakiest wheels so far inside that there are no more. The only important thing right now is to experience whatever you find without judging it or needing to do anything about it.

Yoga Nidra

Our society discourages us from experiencing our bodily sensations but in our bodies is where we find the "controls" for our life energy. The following is a yoga exercise. This exercise will help you become more aware of what is happening inside your body. It is also a means of quick relief from stress. You may want to use a recording or have another person call out the body parts for you as you do this exercise.

Close your eyes. Have someone name a body part. Touch that part with your awareness. Have another body part named and touch it with your awareness. Have your partner continue naming parts of your body, calling out the parts with increasing speed and naming smaller parts until you can no longer keep up.

Another variation of this exercise is to move back and forth between places in your body where you experience opposite feelings. For example, you may move from: tension to relaxation, pain to pleasure, anxiety to ease, depression to excitement or boredom to adventure.

Your body is the most available screen to project your beliefs onto. Any belief, with its emotional charge or attitude, can be experienced in more ways inside yourself than in the outside world. If, for example, you believe that all dogs are vicious as a result of once being bitten by a dog, you will find memories to reinforce this view. You will notice more stories, pictures and movies about vicious dogs. You may possibly find only one personal experience of a dog bite, yet, you have an amazing repertoire of vicious dog thoughts. Perhaps you are not even the one who was bitten, but you felt so much empathy for the bitten person that you created a vicious dog reality with no personal experience. Your imagination can create a false reality. I call it a false reality here but any reality we experience is real and valid to us and we will find aspects of the outside world to reinforce it in our eyes.

As children we are led to believe many things that we will never experience. These are written within, but most of them aren't found in the outside world. Your world within must be larger than your outside world. Your world within is the template through which you experience the outside world. In the instance of the person with the vicious dog belief, it will be nearly impossible for him to experience a friendly dog. His distrust and preconceptions about dogs will cause dogs to distrust and fear him. His feelings will also cause him to actively avoid dogs. He will not be open to a setting where his belief can be changed.

We often get lost in the negative and unpleasant places in our bodies and forget there are as many positive and pleasant places. As you discover the amazing world inside your body, you find that it contains everything that exists outside yourself and more. You can't experience something you don't believe in with senses you don't know you have. All your sensory capabilities start from within your body as your body is the instrument of your sensory experience. Your ability to sense inside is the same as your ability to sense outside. The same is true of your ability to experience. If you haven't found it inside, you cannot find it outside. Your world inside must be larger than your world outside.

Your body is a perfect mirror of how you feel and what you believe at any given time. You can experience this easily. Have a person stand in front of you. Begin to adjust your body so it matches his posture. Ask him any questions that you need to guide you to match posture and attitude. Perhaps ask where he is tense and how much of his weight is on each part of his feet. Have him guide you into his exact posture. As you get closer to matching his posture, notice what you think about and how you feel. Notice the attitude that develops.

Have him think of a situation in which he felt strong emotion. Ask him to guide you in matching the shifts in his body as he brings this memory into awareness. See if you can guess the details of the memory. You will be surprised at the detail that is relayed through another person's body attitude and posture

Personifying the Pain

Personifying the pain is a type of inner child work. I caution you against doing inner child work without the guidance of a professional therapist. This work may evoke traumatic memories and flashbacks.

Bring your awareness to a pain in your body. Gently probe the area with your awareness. Notice the quality of the pain. Is it a burning, itching, tense or tearing pain? Find the epicenter of the pain or where it begins in your body. Begin to trace the pathways of the pain reaching outward in your body. Notice how far from the center of the pain it reaches. Notice the direction, length and shape of the pain. Notice its texture and weight and if it's hard or soft.

Be aware of the feel, shape, size, color and location of the pain. Then personify it on any level of expression. You might ask it to speak to you. Many people find this easy to do. You can talk to the pain as if it were a separate being. Once you are fully aware of the pain, ask it to converse with you in your mind. If this is difficult, ask inside for a part of you to translate for the pain. It may be useful talk out loud to the pain and let it respond out loud. Some questions that might be useful to ask of the pain are:

- Where did you start?
- What do want from or for me?
- What do you need?
- What do you allow me to do that I would not be able to do without you?

These may not be the right questions for you. Be curious. Ask any question that occurs to you. Remember to watch for limiting basic beliefs in the replies such as I am not worthy of living, I deserve pain or disease, I am bad or I have no control over my body or my life.

You can change beliefs by choosing to change them. For example, if you ask a backache what it does for you, you might hear a voice inside your mind reply, "I protect you from people taking advantage of your giving nature."

There are some beliefs that are clear here:

- You feel are a giving person.
- It's hard for you to say no, so you need a way to say no that doesn't make you feel bad about yourself for refusing to help.

- You feel need protection from yourself and other people.
- You feel that people take advantage of you.

This reply gives you several avenues into the belief structure that supports the pain, discomfort or disease. Each limiting belief you change or release helps your overall environment change in a way that contributes to a healthier you. Inner child dialogue is an effective way to work with emotional and belief content. Conflicting beliefs and associated emotions are a source of chronic stress that can inhibit healing on all levels. Another way to think of chronic stress is slow panic.

There are many forms of inner child work and reparenting techniques. Most will work here. Remember that this inner child is you and you must now take over as the parent in this child's life. Treat this child as she needs to be treated, with respect.

Treat this inner child as a younger you who has been hurt and made to feel unacceptable. This child needs to know that she is welcome and lovable. If you find that you cannot accept the child, don't try to force it. It is possible that you are not ready to handle what would emerge. Start with wanting to accept this part of yourself. The guardian aspect of your ego protects you from recognizing what you can't cope with. Respect your own pace.

When you ask inside you may hear something like, "It's like part of me always wants this and another part always wants the opposite." If your inner child has conflicting feelings, the following exercise may be useful.

Imagine that one of the opposing parts is in the palm of one hand and the other part is in the palm of the other hand. You may be interested in the choice of hands you put each image in. Some people think of the left as the feminine or the past and the right as masculine or the future. Ask your inner child what it means to him, if anything. Describe each image in detail and name them if you want. Ask each side to tell his story. After each side clearly presents itself, have the images turn and face each other and start talking to each other. As the conversation progresses, the hands may begin to move closer together. If not, coax them very gently. The object is to get the two images to merge and then place the combined image into your heart. You may want to put the parts in bubbles that merge. Then merge the combined bubble with your heart, or use any other image that appeals to you.

One goal of inner child work is acceptance of the parts of you that you rejected in the past. Self-acceptance causes an effect that is retroactive to the age at which the original trauma occurred. Self-rejection can be the source of many conflicting beliefs and secrets. Once you have accepted a rejected part it will begin to finish its' interrupted developmental process.

Fritz Perls believed in the power of awareness. He believed that if you allow unhindered exploration of any issue, a healthier relationship with it occurs. Always respect all the parts of yourself as if they were separate people. Treat yourself with the same degree of respect you feel would be due to another person. In any situation you may always choose your attitude. When personifying a life challenge you may represent it as an animal, an adult, a child, a part of your higher self, a guide, a mystical being or any other symbol that works for you. Always be flexible with symbols and their interpretation. The only interpretation that is important is your own and it may change. Ask inside to find out the meaning of anything that appears.

Sometimes pain is a sign of healing, change or growth. When you make dramatic changes in your life, you may become afraid and upset. With healing on any level, anxiety, fear, body pain, fever and nausea are common. You must rely on your senses and self-honesty to distinguish between symptoms of healing and symptoms of sickness.

PTSD and Moral Injury

One way to look at PTSD (Post Traumatic Stress Disorder) is to consider it as interrupted trauma that is stuck in your body. The natural shock/trauma process follows an injury. It need not be a physical injury. Shock naturally follows trauma. It immobilizes us until our bodies can recover. If the shock process is not completed there will be a corresponding energetic block in the body until the shock/trauma process is completed. If you bring your awareness to chronic discomforts in your body and hold that awareness without judgment the shock process will complete. Judgment stops the process. You may feel nauseous or dizzy as you release trauma. Relax and let it pass.

Participants and victims of war commonly experience PTSD. One war veteran who was unsuccessfully being treated for PTSD heard the concept of moral injury and knew immediately that this was what he suffered from. The things required of soldiers in war can be an insult to all moral values. It's hard to justify killing another person when your entire upbringing tells you it's wrong. The stress of conflicting beliefs can be debilitating. Mind/body techniques for moral injury are similar to those for PTSD. Settle into your body and bring awareness to discomfort in your body. Keep your awareness with the discomfort without judgment and let its needs unfold. Give yourself what you need to release the trauma and heal.

Love Yourself if You Can

Most of us have parts we feel are unlovable. We also have parts that we love even if we have never acknowledged them. Settle into your body and notice what you are feeling inside right now. Bring your awareness to your feet. Feel your appreciation for your feet and how they help you move in the world. Love your feet if you can. If not, like them and choose to want to love them. If you can't like them, want to like them. Move up your body acknowledging each part of your body and your appreciation for what it does for you. Love the parts if you can. If not like them. If you can't do either, want to like your parts. Include your internal organs. If you feel indifference or hatred or other negative emotions acknowledge them without judgment. Keep moving gently and respectfully toward loving you and all your parts.

Precious Pain

The way we develop our early relationship with pain is easy to see. If you have ever seen a toddler fall and bump his head while his mother is watching you have seen him get up and look to his mother to see how she reacted. If she doesn't pay attention to him, he continues as if nothing much happened. If he sees his mother gasp and hold her breath, he will gasp and hold his breath and begin to cry. Until he learns otherwise, pain is just a sensation of the moment and won't be given much notice unless it's extreme or accompanied by fear.

I remember learning about pain and suffering as a child. At age six, I smashed my finger in a mountain climbing accident. I had to wear a cast on my finger for what seemed like months. The cast was a nuisance, but overall it was not something that held my awareness. The tumble down the mountain, the falling rock and multiple cuts were terrifying to me, but the only real pain I remember was the shot in the rear given by the doctor. Even that was a strange sensation which made one buttock feel heavier than the other.

Not long after the accident I was playing in the yard and an older neighbor boy came up to me and said, "I'll bet you're in a lot of pain."

"Pain?" I replied puzzled. "What's pain?"

I knew hurt, but this pain was different somehow. The neighbor boy, who normally wouldn't talk to me because I was so much younger, explained pain to me and acted like my friend since I had so much of this pain stuff. He taught me that there was virtue in suffering. This changed my relationship with pain completely from a simple signal that something needed attention, that something required suffering. During early childhood is the period of brain development when that portion of the brain which associates with the ability to suffer with pain is becoming fully activated.

Our pain can guide us to maximum health and healing. It may be desirable to reduce pain to a level of comfort that allows you to be functional and open to its guidance. If you break your leg, some pain is useful to remind you that you have a serious injury and need to allow ample time for healing. If you had no pain, you would probably not take care of yourself or allow yourself to heal properly. Your leg might even deteriorate to the point where you would never be able to walk normally again. Even small, subtle pain can tell you something and lead you to healing a part of your life.

We may confuse pain with suffering. Although they often occur at the same time, one has little to do with the other. Pain is a simple sensory signal of the state of your body or emotions. The part of your brain that processes physical pain is the same part that processes emotional pain. All emotional pain has a physical aspect and all physical pain has an emotional aspect. To the brain the two are the same. One study indicated that emotional pain could be treated with Tylenol. Awareness must be brought to the pain to separate the physical from the emotional. Suffering is the verbal and emotional process we go through when we are in pain.

If you simply keep your awareness with any pain sensation, taking the role of an objective, impersonal observer, the larger aspects of the sensation will begin to present themselves. These sensations might be pain, itching, tickling, muscle tightness or any other bodily sensations. Mercy, the lack of judgment, is essential. Self-judgment can be pathological, eating away at our emotions, causing chronic low level stress, creating an environment friendly to physical and mental health problems.

One effective route to healing, or changing, a part of your life is to intend the change and bring awareness to your body. The feelings and other awareness in your body provides a reliable guide to your unique healing needs. Mindfulness meditations, or being present with your body, have been shown to benefit health in many ways even causing changes in the expression of genes. One study found that various mindfulness meditations caused genes associated with inflammation to down-regulated. DNA is expressed by the strength of each genes expression. Some genes are expressed at a higher strength than others. Expressing genes associated with a disease results in development of the disease. Turning down the strength of these genes causes the disease to cease. One way of looking at it is that when cancer genes are expressed at a high strength we bloom with cancer. When the genes are·expressed at low strength the cancer goes into remission.

Because of the construction of the human brain, emotional and physical pain are hard to separable. According to the triune brain theory, one way to look at brain development and function, the human brain is made up of three main levels or brains. The job of the brain stem or reptilian complex is to maintain basic life support, sexual drive and to tell us to run from danger. The awareness of the reptilian brain is limited to the physical world of daily survival and yet all nerve circuitry to higher brain levels passes through the brain stem. If the emotional affairs of the old mammalian brain, the next area of higher development and function, cause pain, that pain is detected by the brain stem and represented in the only way possible as physical pain to run away from.

Any physical pain you feel has a counterpart in emotions and reason. Reason is the realm of the next higher brain complex, the neo-mammalian brain. Even if a wound is purely physical, such as a broken leg, there is also an emotional wound. You may feel stupid for having followed the ski patrol through terrain you weren't skilled enough to be on and humiliated when they had to bring you down the mountain on a stretcher, or just terrified to see and feel your broken bone. This is certainly emotional pain.

To soothe the emotional pain that compounds the physical pain, you may try telling yourself that it's all the fault of the snow groomers who neglected to cover the rock you hit, consequently, breaking your leg. This compounds the pain again by adding the psychological pain of blaming someone else and thereby choosing to be a victim.

You might react to the psychological pain by choosing the belief that you are inadequate, and it is therefore God's fault that you broke your leg. God must not love you, so you react in anger - now adding spiritual pain, the realm of the next higher brain complex, sometimes referred to as the angle brain.

Moral injury can also play a role. If you are wounded in a war where you observed and maybe participated in actions that violated your moral values, healing may be inhibited by the associated beliefs and resulting emotional charges. Being a soldier can require you to do things you believe are wrong because your government tells you to. You may justify these actions, but there may always be a part of you the feels that you have done wrong. Moral injury, like emotional injury, can inhibit healing.

There is no separation in this process. All levels of involvement occur at the same time. The different ways the layers of your brain are able to represent the world are some of the different ways that you naturally represent your world to yourself. You may approach healing on any of these levels.

With an emotional charge there is a belief that supports it. If the emotional charge is the need for love, the accompanying belief might be, I am not lovable or there is no love available for me. Pain works the same way. To discover the emotional, physical, mental and spiritual aspects of pain, keep your awareness with the pain long enough to allow it to reveal itself. If you have judgments about the pain or yourself for having the pain, you will probably block yourself from having the clarity to discover more about it. In some cases, the pain represents a part of yourself you don't accept. By itself, nonjudgmental acceptance of the pain will take you far in your healing. It's important to note that acceptance is not the same as giving up. Acceptance is the practical action of honestly assessing where you are right now and what you need to do to get where you want to be.

Dance with Pain

Touching any life challenge can cause an increase in blood flow and oxygenation to the associated part of your body. Healing assets such as white blood cells and stem cells can be increased by increasing awareness and intent to heal. If pain is overwhelming, increasing awareness may increase the pain and associated stress and distress producing the opposite of the desired outcome.

When pain is substantial, adjust your healing tactics. Imagine a situation where your life challenge is healed and you are enjoying the result. For example, if you have a torn ligament in your knee the pain may be extreme. You might imagine with as many senses as possible that you are running, skiing, playing or doing what you enjoy most that requires strong and functioning knees. Feel the joy of the activity. When the experience is strong in your inner senses touch your knee with awareness. Bring the joy of the activity into your knee. When the pain gets intense move back into the activity. Move back and forth between the activity and the pain until the pain has subsided enough to work deeply and directly in it with your senses. When you send the intent to heal to a part of your body (or a part of your life) you increase healing activity. This works for emotional pain as well.

There are many techniques to turn down the pain to make it easier to work with. You might use the image of pain being tied to a dimmer switch or volume control. It might be helpful to move away with your awareness like observing from outside your body. In all healing what works best is what's most natural for you.

Healing Without Content

Using metaphors or imagery is often helpful in healing but there are times when a wordless, imageless delivery of intent is useful and may be more efficient. Mindfulness meditation is the practice of simply being aware and present with what is happening here and now. This practice has been shown to switch genes on or off or to vary the intensity of gene expression to create improved health. This is a way of working pre-verbally with your life challenge, or without content. You may experience catharsis or shock and have no idea why, but you still gain the same benefit as discovering the story of the trauma and reframing it to create a healthier relationship with it. You can bring your awareness to any life challenge and give it the quality of energy (awareness) that it needs without words. You can continue to direct this energy, without describing it or your life challenge, to your life challenge until it is healed. As you change your energy body the rest of your world automatically adjusts.

Inspection Tour

I invite you to go on a tour of your body. On this tour, if you find anything that doesn't feel right, that isn't getting proper nourishment, which needs repair, increased waste disposal or anything else, you can create helpers to keep the work in progress as you continue. These helpers can call on any other part of your body to nurture the healing process. They can call for support from other parts of your body. There's a greater consciousness inside that knows how to heal. You can trust your inner guidance to find your own healing. Healing and cure are very different things. Only you can decide what healing means to you. And the most reliable guide, to finding that healing and making it your own, is the guidance you find inside. So I invite you to trust that guidance as we begin this journey.

Begin this inspection with your skin. Your skin is the largest organ of your body and the most sensitive. Your skin contains you and keeps you from leaking out. It also protects you by letting in what you need to nourish you, yet, it keeps out things that can harm you. Your skin is a membrane and it can choose what to let in and what to let out.

A lot of waste is washed out through your skin and yet the water can't penetrate it to get inside your body. Your skin is waterproof. Scan your skin with your awareness and notice how well it's containing you, how well it's protecting you. Are you too thin skinned? Do physical, emotional or energetic toxins get through your skin? Do you leak outward? Is your skin too thick? So thick that it doesn't allow the nourishment in or the toxins to escape? If there are places where your skin leaks, leave some helpers to make repairs. If your skin feels too thin send out workers to make your skin thicker. If it's too thick have them make it thinner. Do whatever feels right. You're the one in your body. Use your senses to discover what's right for you.

Leave your helpers in charge of the various projects working with your skin. Continue now to your bones. Your skeletal system is the hardest part of your body. It's what makes it possible for you to stand up. And yet your bones are not really that solid. They're constantly changing. Notice if your bones are hard and shiny on the outside. Are they thick enough? Are they getting the nutrition they need? If not, send out messages to the proper places in your body to obtain the nutrition you need for your bones. Increase appetite for foods that provide the nutrients you need. Notice if your skeleton feels connected, like a single unit. Is your bone marrow healthy? Is it receiving all the materials it needs to perform its functions, like building white blood cells and stem cells? And are the waste products being properly washed away. If there's anything to be improved, go ahead and create or dispatch any helpers needed to carry on the work while you continue to your muscles.

Scan your muscles. Notice any places that they might be stressed or damaged. Begin repairs in those places. Notice if they're in proper working condition. Are they properly exercised? Are they getting proper nutrition? Are they getting enough blood? Are the wastes being washed away? Are they tense or relaxed? Are there any knots in your muscles? Do they have what they need to build new muscle? Are they coordinating properly with your nervous system and your sensory systems? Begin whatever repairs are needed. If they're not getting enough blood, increase the blood flow. Clean out the blood vessels. Increase oxygenation. Increase appetite for the foods you need for proper nutrition and elimination. Increase appetite for fun physical exercise. Whatever's needed, just do it.

Bring your awareness to your heart. Is it clean and healthy? Is it damaged? Is it clogged? Whatever needs to be done, begin the work? Create the necessary helpers. Follow the blood throughout your body. Is your blood healthy? Does it have everything it needs? Is it being properly cleaned? Is it getting enough oxygen from your lungs and giving enough oxygen to the rest of the body? Is it performing all its functions properly? Whatever's needed, send out your workers to do it. Order the creation of the necessary workers if they are not available and move on.

Bring your awareness to your lungs. Are they working properly? Are they exchanging oxygen and waste gases properly? Are they in good repair? Are they soft and supple? Whatever is needed here just go ahead and do it and move to your kidneys. Are they working properly, removing wastes from your body? Are they working in harmony with your glands? And are your hormones working in harmony with the rest of your body? Are your glands swollen? Cleanse any impurities from your glands. Whatever's needed, do it now and move from your lymphatic system to your nervous system.

Are your neural pathways clear so that information can pass freely? Are the nerve endings clear, clean and alive? Is there damage? Is the insulation cracked or missing? Are the nerve endings healthy?

Notice how your nervous system connects your brain with the rest of your body. It's as if the nerve endings are the controls that operate your body and your brain is your onboard computer. Notice how all this is working. There's no need to understand how, or why, your body works? All you need to do is create the helpers with the intent that they adjust or repair any part of your body or mind. Trust your own abilities to bring balance that creates the condition that is health for you. You know what feels right in your own body. Create your helpers as needed and set the process in motion.

Bring your awareness to your mouth and notice that starting at your mouth there's a tunnel that goes all the way through your body and even though it's inside your body, it's also outside your body. As things pass through this tunnel your body takes what it needs to nourish it. Then, it lets what it doesn't need pass on through to be washed away, to be carried away in your daily eliminations. Bring your awareness to your mouth and notice if everything is working properly. If it isn't, begin repairs before you move on to your throat and then to your stomach. Notice if the proper chemicals, in the proper balances, and enough water, are available for proper digestion. Notice if the needed nutrients are being extracted from your food and properly absorbed.

Notice any damage. Whatever you find, take the proper action to move toward better health. Move through your small intestines. Notice any repairs, or improvements, needed and order any needed work to begin. Move on through your large intestine. If any repairs are needed, or if balances need adjusting, set the process in motion and move on. Notice your organs of elimination, your bladder, colon, rectum and anus. If anything isn't working right, or anything is in need of adjustment, call on your healing assets to do whatever is needed and move on.

Move to your sexual organs. If there's anything that needs to be done here initiate the process and move on.

Check your sinuses and ears, your sensory capabilities and any other part of your body that has been overlooked. Take all the time you need to go back through your body to inventory the changes you have chosen. Double check with your workers to be certain there are no misunderstandings of your intent. Take all the time you need. When you're ready, allow your eyes to open and your consciousness to return to the room around you.

CHAPTER 4
EXERCISE WITH NO PAIN - CONSTANT GAIN

I Love Recess

I was 49-years-old and told I might die any moment from a heart attack or stroke as the result of extreme sleep apnea. I only breathed for 20 minutes out of an hour when I was asleep. My heart rate and blood oxygen levels would drop to dangerous levels every night. As it progressed my hands and feet went numb. My muscles burned constantly from lack of oxygen. My organs were shutting down and it actually hurt to think. I could only stay awake for about 20 minutes at a time at its worst point. Up to that time I didn't know what was causing my health problems and could not find an effective way to deal with them. With the knowledge that came with finally knowing what I was facing I was able to heal.

I did a treadmill stress test and had to stop after less than 3 minutes out of fatigue. I was told that I was in average condition for a man my age. This made me aware that I badly needed physical exercise as part of my healing treatment. Along with meditation, toning and chanting, I used exercise to cure my apnea. After one month of taking control of my healing process I did another sleep study and was declared to have only borderline apnea with no need for treatment. I learned to approach exercise as play and as a way to free the part of me that was afraid to have fun or play.

I needed the jubilant child part of me, the part that knew how to play, to participate to be successful in long-term exercise. Where I grew up acting joyful brought quick attack. A jubilant child would have been met with comments such as, "There's something wrong with that kid". The parents of the child would've been embarrassed at the behavior. If it continued the child might have been shunned for fear that such behavior was contagious. It would not be easy to revive the playful part in me, if one had ever existed.

When I thought about the jubilant child, who may have existed in me, I saw a small, scared boy sitting alone on a playground. He didn't want to look up for fear that making eye contact would constitute some kind of breach of etiquette that would make him even more unacceptable. This child was subjected to constant severe judgment.

He knew because he was the keeper of the self-judgment, the one who was swift to self-punishment for violation of social rules never spoken. The rules must be figured out according to a seemingly brutal withholding of love by those whose lives children rely on. These rules that are never really explained, are constructed as well as possible in the mind of the child who lacks the presumptive concepts of social relationships. They can hold terrible rein over a child's ability to develop and thrive in the world. And yet it's we ourselves who impose these misinformed boundaries on ourselves in an effort to be good children.

In order to free this lonely frightened boy who held the key to my jubilance, and therefore possibly to my life, I would need to gain his trust. Even though this boy was me, he had no reason to trust me. I/he was the one who had emotionally brutalized this child.

I started out with a single minute of exercise, walking on the treadmill as slowly as it would move, keeping all thoughts from my mind and my awareness on making it safe for the jubilant child to emerge and to play. When I was able to be totally present with the child for a full minute I earned another minute and was able to go for two minutes the next day. When I could totally let that child takeover for two minutes I earned another minute. Each minute of creating a safe environment and being present with the child earned another minute. If I violated the child's trust by allowing unsafe thoughts or by not being present with the child, I had to start over again at one minute.

As I progressed, my walk became a dance and I began to look forward to my exercise time. I use the Tai Chi approach of 1 inch and one pebble at a time. There are legendary Tai Chi masters called leapers. Leapers can jump to great heights and perform amazing aerial acrobatics. They learn to do this by digging a hole 1 inch deep and jumping out of it. When they can do this with ease, they dig the whole another inch deeper and put a pebble in a pocket. Over the years becomes very deep and the weight of the pebbles very heavy. Each inch and each pebble is earned by developing the strength and grace to leap from the hole with ease.

With each new minute of exercise that I earned I added a little weight to my body and increased the speed and incline on the treadmill. As I gained trust and became more acquainted with my jubilant child I began to see subtle changes in my life. I started feeling friendlier and less distrustful of people I encountered. My energy level increased and my apnea virtually disappeared. My body has slowly and steadily transformed. The jubilant child grew to be a jubilant man as I provided the safety he needed to thrive.

Over the past 12 years I have used treadmill: running backwards, forward, sideways and in circles while using hand, wrist, ankle and body weights; ellipse: using weights and going backward and forward; free weights; weight machine; light hand weights and aerobic dance. I used to have body envy during the Olympic Games looking at the young athletes but for the past two Olympics the athlete's bodies looked like mine. At over 60-years-old I have the best looking body of my entire life. I'm 13 years, at the time of this writing, into a 30 year plan to play my way to constantly improving physical and mental health. I'm convinced that our bodies will do whatever we demand of them. If we choose to sit around and become old our bodies will oblige. If we decide to run a marathon our bodies will rise to the occasion with proper training regardless of age. If we choose to exercise our bodies in a playful, healthy way, making each session more fun, adding more flexibility movements, endurance and strength moves each day, our bodies will respond by growing stronger and more flexible.

We tend to want to make things happen instantly. If exercise is approached with this attitude you will probably fail to make it a daily part of your life that you look forward to and love to do. More likely you will get very sore and quit. Unless you're training for an athletic event take your time and grow enough each day that you feel no pain, or very little pain. I've actually come to like a small amount of muscle pain of the good kind that comes from working muscles. It lets me know I'm making progress. I'm building a body to dependably carry me through a century of life with ease, able to do the tasks that I might encounter. I am not training to be an athlete or warrior. I play accordingly.

I knew before I started exercising that the no pain - no gain model wouldn't work for me. A Harvard study showed that how you feel about exercise influences the benefits you receive from it. Work equals drudgery to many people. A workout is just more drudgery. I saw people my whole life who started doing things requiring physical effort with such gusto that within a few days they were so stiff and sore that they never did it again. I chose to exercise with an attitude of play allowing a maximum work out time rather than the typical minimum. I also chose to use the Tai Chi one inch and one pebble at a time approach. When I earned another minute of trust from my jubilant inner child I made my exercise a little harder increasing one or more: weight; speed; incline; agility; impact and resistance. And more important, I made it more fun every day and kept it safe for my inner child to express himself.

A typical workout (recess) will start with me standing with eyes closed and taking a few deep breaths. I settle deeply into my body bringing my awareness to my feet and letting it rise through the rest of my body until I am aware of my entire body as a unit. I begin to move very gently with small, relaxed motions feeling what's happening inside. I notice aches, pains and stiffness. I let the part of my body that calls the loudest direct the movement. Movements are always as relaxed as possible and done very slowly at first. It actually takes more strength and balance to move slowly. The slower you move the more speed, core strength and flexibility you build. If you can make a movement very slowly it is unlikely that you will hurt yourself performing the move at normal speeds.

If it's your first time using this technique, it's time to quit for the day after one minute. You have used up your first minute. If you were able to do the first minute with a relaxed body, staying present in your mind, without judgmental words in your head, respecting your jubilant inner child, then you have earned another minute. Adding one minute at a time may seem like it will take forever to get in shape, or to even see results, but it adds up quickly. It takes very little exercise to feel some benefit.

Everything in this approach is guided by your body and what it needs now. Over time you'll begin to notice what your body wants and doesn't want and honoring it will become natural. This may reach into all areas of your health guiding you to enjoy a healthier way of eating, learning to honor the needs and guidance of your body, mind and spirit. It seems simple but in our society we tend to learn to feel as little as possible ignoring the richness of our emotions and physical senses.

With each minute you earn add something to make your exercise more challenging and more suited to your needs. If you are training for a marathon your needs are different than the average person who wants to be able to do the things required in their lives with ease and grace. A marathon runner may need to run many miles to prepare. An average person may find building agility, balance, strength and endurance by dancing in small circles with light weights, or using a balance ball, or any other exercise technique or device, is appropriate.

I always use music because it adds rhythm to my exercise and makes the time fly and the movement fun. Choose music that feels right to you at the moment. I have used every kind of music to exercise at different times. What works best is what is the most fun.

Notice that you feel different music in different parts of your body. Music that you feel in the part of your body you're working on seems to add more stimulation and awareness to the area. Brain scan and MRI technology show that if you think about a part of your body blood flow will increase to that part. If you're healing a part of your body bringing your awareness to that part will increase healing speed. If you are building muscle, Arnold Schwarzenegger said that one rep with visualization is worth 10 without. Any way you increase your awareness of a body part will increase the energy flow there.

Western people tend to do better with meditation and visualization that involves movement. Experiment while you exercise with visualizations that clean out deposits of toxins and wastes, or strengthen or rebuild weak or injured parts, clean and heal organs, build new muscles and blood vessels, connect with spiritual realms, work with body energy or anything else that appeals to you. You can use any of the exercises, or visualizations, presented here to enhance your exercise. Adjust them to fit your needs. Meditations that silently bring awareness to different parts of your body, or aspects of you, can be very useful in healing and in building a stronger body. Energy normally wasted on words is channeled to more productive uses when we work on a non-verbal, or pre-verbal level. Running words through our minds uses a lot of energy. Most of us are familiar with wasting more energy thinking about doing a task than it actually takes to get up and do the task. Try turning down your inner dialogue and turning up your sensory awareness while exercising.

Dancing with Weights

When I first started exercising, I mainly used a treadmill. I would start as slow as the treadmill would go. I always begin by moving as slowly as I can while staying relaxed. I use very slow movements to be sure I don't hurt myself as well. If I can do a move, or lift a weight in a particular way, while moving as slow as possible and keeping relaxed as I move, I believe it won't hurt me to do it faster, or with more weight.

At first I only walked and ran on the treadmill going forward. When I heard about someone using light weights while walking on a treadmill I decided to try it and I like it a lot. Every day I added a little weight to my wrists, ankles or waist, or increased the incline, length of time, or intensity of my sessions. Of course, every day I worked to make it more fun as well.

After about a year and a half I was running up steep inclines at fairly high speed with ever increasing amounts of time while packing up to 60 lbs of weights on my body. My hamstrings got very tight and very uncomfortable. Nothing I could do would relax them. I went to a chiropractor who was the nearest to my house. That was a bad decision. I called the chiropractor, Sledge Hammer, because if your only tool is a hammer you see every problem as something to pound. He had no idea how to deal with this condition and instead of researching it, or asking for advice, he tore the ligament that holds my left hip socket together so every time I moved wrong it felt as if a dagger were stabbing into my hip. Had he, or I, researched the problem, a quick web search revealed that I was experiencing a condition common in tri-athletes that is easily and quickly treated with massage or acupuncture. Sledge Hammer shared an office with both kinds of practitioners. Nine years later I still find myself awake in the middle of the night because of pain from my chiropractic injury.

I learned a few things from this experience. I learned that when I don't take responsibility for my own healing things don't go as well as they might. I also learned that flexibility is as important as strength and endurance. When I was able to get back on the treadmill I ran sideways, backward and in circles as well as forward. I have not been able to rebuild the strength I had before. I am limited by the strength of the ligament, but I followed my body's signals and learned to work around it as it healed.

I found an exercise ball very helpful when I was limited in movement and body part involvement due to injury. It allowed me stretch isolated muscles without reinjuring myself. I started with very short movements advancing to long movements rolling on the balls surface. Movements were always slow and relaxed. The ball allowed me to build core strength and balance while protecting the injured part of my body.

One of my favorite forms of exercise is aerobics with light weights. I call it dancing with weights because I have fun doing it. I put on music that stimulates the part of my body that I am working on. Most days I use music that I feel in pelvic and core muscles. I begin my exercise session standing with my eyes closed holding light weights starting with 1 lb. I settle into my body feeling myself dropping into my feet and filling the rest of my body with awareness as I move upward.

When I have settled into my body I begin to sway moving the weights slightly. I feel my whole body and bring my awareness to any part that is sore or painful or stiff. Whatever part calls out the loudest become the center of movement following my body's senses to move in a way that gives the part what it needs. The pain, stiffness, or restriction of movement usually subsides. When the part is no longer the loudest I move to the next loudest part to give the part what it needs. It may need flexibility, stretching, increased blood/oxygen flow, strengthening, sound or something else. As I move from one part to another the intensity and speed increase. I slowly move up in weights from 1 lb., to 2 lb., to 3 lb., to 5 lb., to 8 lb., to 10 lb., to 12 lb., to 15 lb. I may not go through all the weights. I may also start with 3 lbs instead of 1. Do what's right for you in the moment as you let your body guide you.

Breathing is very important. You can make good progress toward improved overall health by doing only breathing exercises. Breathing into different parts of your body directs your awareness to that part and this alone will increase blood flow. Try breathing deeply while you exercise, adding a shout, grunt, or chant to make it even deeper and bring awareness more intently to the part you are working on. Experiment with different breaths. Try shallow breathing, making silly sounds with your breath, inhaling as your abdomen contracts and exhaling as it expands, or any other pattern that occurs to you. As you play you will discover what works for you. The more breath you direct to a part the more productive your play will be. This is a way of visualizing.

The more blood and oxygen you have flowing to a body part, the more healing function you have in that part of your body.

While exercising, or playing, there is only one movement, one step, one lift, one jump or one anything. That is the one you are doing now. Movements from the past no longer matter. Movements in the future are not yet happening. If you keep your mind focused on the movement you make now, you will be amazed at how much more endurance you have and how quickly your allotted time passes.

It takes only a little weight to reap benefits of resistance training. You can lift 100 lbs a few times but not get the overall benefit that you will get from lifting 1 lb. a hundred times. The most important aspect of dancing with weights is to have fun. Keep present and play with increasing jubilance and you will find yourself feeling younger and stronger daily.

As we age our eyes get slower and less flexible. One way to counter this is to constantly move your gaze focusing on small objects as quickly as you can while exercising. Reading the smallest print you can also help. Like the rest of our bodies, our eyes will adapt to level of activity we demand of them.

Aspirin

As the result of the chiropractic injury above I had to deal with constant pain for several years. I found that aspirin worked best for me. I took the pills according to bottle direction, never exceeding recommended doses. After a few months I began to get what felt like small muscles tears in my hands, biceps and arches when I exercised that got progressively worse with time. It seemed like every exercise session would cause new tears. Aspirin would take the pain away quickly. I thought it was a miracle drug.

One day I came home from work and my wife wanted to talk about her day. I went directly to the aspirin bottle and took two. I said, "Just give me a minute until the aspirin kicks in." To me it sounded too much like, "Just a minute until the alcohol kicks in." It made me think that there was more happening with me and aspirin than I was realizing. I looked up the side effects of aspirin and found that it breaks down muscle fiber. I was taking this substance for the pain that was mainly caused by the damage the substance was doing to my body. It took away the pain that it caused. It was true addiction.

I talked to a doctor about it. He said he'd never heard of that reaction. He also admitted that in his 30 years as a doctor he had prescribed aspirin many times, yet had never read the side effects. He found it hard to believe that aspirin was actually causing my muscle tears, but I quit using aspirin and quit tearing muscles. His education didn't include aspirin side effects so he couldn't imagine it being important. The information provided to medical professionals by pharmaceutical companies was found to be more than 80% marketing information and only 12% actual data in a recent study. My body awareness said it was a harmful substance if used daily. I followed my awareness and corrected the problem.

Breath

Many cultures consider breath as life force. Some names are: life energy, healing energy, prana, chi, ki, and Shakti. In Yoga the breath is central to all life, health and healing. The health benefits of deep breathing are obvious, but breath is also a powerful envelope, or tool, for stimulating the healing process by delivering it to specific areas of the body. Breathing exercises also bring greater body awareness and increased mental clarity fortify intention and awareness.

Breathing Exercises

There are thousands of breathing techniques. Any exercise that allows you to safely increase your breathing volume is probably beneficial to your physical health and self-awareness, however there are medical reasons for some people to refrain from doing exercises that involve deep breathing. If you believe you might be such a person consult your physician before doing this or any other breathing exercise. Breathing can be a powerful catalyst for moving old, stuck emotions. Some breathing patterns can cause disorientation and even hallucination. If you experience distressing results, use the awareness to avoid that unhealthy breathing style in your daily life. Use negative experiences as learning resources. If you are emotionally unstable, only do deep breathing exercises with the supervision of an appropriate teacher or therapist.

Settle into a comfortable position either sitting or lying down, it makes no difference. Notice how you breathe. How deeply are you breathing? Does your breath only move in your upper chest, in and out, or is it moving in your belly as well? Are you breathing deep into your abdomen? Notice where you are right at this moment. Notice the quality of your breathing as the air moves in and out through your sinuses, down the back of your throat into your lungs and back out again. Is it easy or labored, clear or restricted? Allow your breath to move a little deeper into your belly, breathing a little deeper. Increase the volume of air moving in and out of your lungs. Allowing your breathing to drop a little deeper into your pelvic floor.

Imagine that attached to your tailbone and pubic bone are the handles of a bellows. Each time you inhale the handles move apart, drawing air into your lungs. Feel the bellows pulling air deep into your lungs and into your abdomen, drawing it right down to your pelvic floor. Squeeze the air out as completely as possible from the bottom of your lungs upward. Experience your breath as it flows in and out of your body. Inhale deeply into your abdomen, deeper with each breath. And as you exhale begin to imagine that your breath moves up from your pelvic floor, up through your spine and out the top of your head cascading down around you in all directions, enveloping you in a cocoon of breath. Inhale deeply into your lungs and as you exhale imagine your breath moving through the core of your body, out through the top of your head, cascading down around you then coming back up through the bottoms of your feet, through your pelvic floor, back up through the core of your body and out through the top of your head in a continuous stream of breath. Imagine your breath flowing around you like a living shell of breath. Take as much time as you like to experience this cocoon of breath as it moves around you and through you, nurturing and protecting you. When you're ready, allow your awareness to gently return to the room around you.

Sound

Physicists say all matter contains the essential energy of the universe and is held in a solid state by sound vibration. Light exists in the energy matter continuum between energy and matter. All sound is energy. All light is energy and sound. All matter is energy, sound and light. All sound carries an innate rhythm and frequency. The rhythm and frequency create harmony, or disharmony, with our internal and external environments. We each have our own unique innate sounds and rhythms that interact internally and externally harmoniously or disharmoniously. We are super complex instruments playing in a symphony of life. This is a symphony of personal life, family life, extended family life, global life and spiritual life. Each symphony plays within a larger symphony on into infinity. In this sense, we are all master musicians. We contribute to and have influence over the pulse and harmony of the universe. We can choose harmony or disharmony.

We have an innate ability to use the therapeutic aspects of sound with our bodies guiding us. When we have a headache, we may naturally make an ahhhh or an oooo sound. These soothing vowel sounds massage the brain and inside the head and neck. When you have a headache, you would never want to make, or hear, a piercing eeee sounds. This may be a useful sound for constipation, or for breaking up other restrictions, but you would find it hard to even think this sound when you have a splitting headache. Your body will guide you in the use of sound. Trust it.

There are many electronic sound devices available for healing. These are probably unnecessary. You can probably produce any sound necessary with little risk of self-generated sound causing harm. The safety factor in using sound that you generate yourself is the fact that you can constantly monitor and control the sound according to what you feel in response to the sound.

If a sound feels good to your body, it is a safe bet that the particular sound at the present intensity is not harmful and probably beneficial. If it hurts to make a sound, stop making it. If you get overly jubilant, you may risk strained vocal chords, but this is probably not serious in the absence of any medical problem with your throat, vocal chords or other body parts involved in making sound.

Noxious sound bombards us daily with constant, subtle stress. There are sirens, trucks, airplanes, jackhammers, computer hum, fluorescent light buzz, refrigerators, screaming children and music we don't like. It's interesting that toxicity of a sound, in most cases, is how we feel about it. Studies show that the most healing music in hospitals is the music you like. Many adults find Mozart's music is soothing and healing, but they usually find heavy metal music to be irritating and a hindrance to healing. For adolescents the opposite may be true.

The sources of noxious sound are almost endless. We can counter these noise by a process similar to the inner workings of sound cancelling car mufflers. As the engine exhaust passes through the exhaust pipe, a computer analyzes the sound and a cancelling sound plays through tiny speakers in the exhaust pipe. The result of the two sounds together is almost no exhaust noise. Similarly, we can drown out noxious noise by humming or singing sounds that that counter it.

The work of French physician A. A. Tomatis suggests that most of the sound needed to maintain good listening or promote better healing is found in Gregorian chants. He found that Gregorian Monks were sick and unable to cope with the energy demands of their lifestyle if they were deprived the several hours of chanting that is part of their normal day. Their health and vigor returned quickly when chanting was restored to their daily routines.

Toning

The easiest way to develop a sense of what sound does inside your body is an exercise called toning. To begin make any elongated vowel sound and see how it feels. Notice which parts of your body absorb or resonate with the sound. Notice which tones soothe and which tones irritate. Spend five to ten minutes a day doing this exercise and you will soon find many new uses for self-generated sound. You will probably feel better, have more energy and find your mind is sharper.

When working with sound, allow your body to guide you. Quiet yourself inside and become grounded. Bring your awareness to a life challenge. The life challenge may be anything, even something as small as a slightly tensed muscle. As you probe inside, you will find something to work on even if you can think of nothing that needs healing. Allow whatever sound that occurs to come out. As you continue, the clarity of the life challenge (physical, emotional, belief or energetic) increases and the clarity of the sound quality increases. Your sensory feedback guides you in all aspects.

Toning has been particularly useful in remapping neural pathways by stimulating a path from the area of bodily disorder to the brain. Toning does not overlook other forms of self-generated sound such as singing, whistling, chanting and yodeling. Using a musical instrument to sound your life challenge is also effective. Use whatever feels right for you.

CHAPTER 5
TECHNIQUES

In the practice of mind/body healing, a variety of practical techniques are available. The Taoist Priests have compiled more than twelve hundred volumes of writings on qigong, an ancient system that uses visualization. There are many good books on mind/body healing, but the most effective techniques are those that are natural to you and easy for you to use. Use your own senses and inner guidance to find what works best for you in your situation. Be creative and have fun and use humor in your healing practice.

Sensitivity Cycle

Ron Kurtz in Body-Centered Psychotherapy, The Hakomi Method describes the process of awareness and intent in daily life as the Sensitivity Cycle. He says that, first, there is a stage of relaxation where you drop your outside world view and begin to reorient to your internal needs. You notice what you need, or want, now and follow your innate guidance to fulfillment. For example, you relax and realize that you are hungry. You check inside and find that you are hungry for rice and beans, not cake.

Next comes effective action. You're aware of what your body needs, you have identified what is necessary to fill that need and now you act to get it. When you have eaten the rice and beans, you have reached satisfaction, the last stage of the sensitivity cycle. Now you may relax, reorient to what you now need, or want, and start the cycle again. If you fail to complete any of the stages, hunger and nourishment aren't satisfied, and you become stuck in that stage until it is satisfied.

In the physical healing process we see the same dynamics. The metaphoric and sensory symbolic language of the unconscious mind has become fairly well-defined by modern behavioral science and provides a channel of communication between our physical maladies and our conscious minds. Each person relates to the world with a unique blend of symbolism that includes sound, vision, speech, emotion and bodily sensations. Using our own symbolism, it's easier to choose a new intent and continue the sensitivity cycle toward our own healing.

For example, if a person has trouble with anger and blanks out language then only sees the red light of rage, it is better to focus on seeing the redness of rage than to talk about the virtue of not losing your temper. Stepping into the experience makes its attributes available now.

Most people require some form of symbolism, at first, to deliver the intent and to process the awareness or innate guidance. The symbols help to maintain concentration and focus. The symbolic form makes no difference. A person may be naturally more inclined to imagery, meditation, sound, movement, feeling or other methods. All symbols are the result of preverbal experience and as such always reflect the vibrational truth of our state of being. What we experience is registered truthfully and accurately while being presented in different symbols. It's when we translate experience into words that we rapidly lose truth and accuracy. As you learn to move farther away from the verbal description of the event to the actual experience, you become more accustomed to being present instead of two steps removed from the event.

When you work with imagery, in the language of Milton Erickson, MD, you are in essence accessing resource states. For example, if in a hypnotic state you are given the suggestion that wind is blowing through a wart on your hand, the image will probably cause an increase in blood oxygen to the area of the wart. The wart may begin to disappear if you are not unconsciously hanging onto the wart because of a belief such as I am ugly and deserve to have warts. Of course this belief, like all beliefs, has an emotional charge that goes along with it that may cause chronic low level stress resulting in the decreased blood flow and oxygenation that allow a wart. The belief you are ugly may create the stress the wart requires. Releasing the emotional charge changes the environment so it is no longer is conducive to warts.

If you have been caught in a tornado and are terrified of wind, the suggestion of wind blowing through you might cause the opposite effect by contracting the muscles and decreasing the oxygen in the area of the wart. In each case the way you hold your life energy is different. Energy always follows thought; physical form follows energetic form. Kirlian photography shows that before a plant grows a new leaf the energetic outline of the leaf appears and then the energy field fills into the actual leaf.

The gentle, healing wind in the first example brings a useful resource state. The tornado brings a counterproductive state.

You can change your energy, energy being a precursor to matter, in the environment of the wart by simply bringing awareness to it with the intent that it go away. If there is an overwhelming emotional charge and the real intent toward this wart is that it exist, it won't go away. It isn't easy to give up your defenses unquestioned.

The use of imagery is the use of intent and awareness. When you intend an outcome, you begin to become aware of the situation and the possible action which you need to take to create the outcome. If you take effective action, you move closer to your goal. If you take an ineffective action, you learn it doesn't work and you move on to another plan of action always bringing you closer to your goal. Your intent takes you to possible actions. Within the action is the intent. The intent becomes the guidance that brings the awareness of the need to change the plan of action or intent. Intent and awareness aren't separate events or entities. They are the two sides of the flipping coin and cannot exist separately.

Relaxation

One of the most powerful techniques to promote good health and healing of any life challenge is simple relaxation. An amazing amount of tension exists in most people's bodies as they go through their daily lives. Tension can come from many sources. Relaxing the tensions in your body relaxes the tensions in your mind.

Lie on your back on the floor, if possible, otherwise any comfortable position will do. Take some deep, slow breaths as you settle into your body. Notice what your body feels. Many people are unable to feel their bodies most of the time resulting from cultural training that teaches us that our bodies are bad and the feelings inside are to be ignored. There are many ways that we learn to avoid feeling our bodies. I spent many years of my life floating above my body where I didn't have to feel. If it's difficult for you to feel what's happening in your body, go slowly and respect yourself.

Bring your awareness to your toes. Feel your breath moving through your body parts as you relax them. Use whatever method you choose and relax your toes. Move slowly up your body relaxing muscles as completely as possible as you go. Take time to relax the small muscles in your feet. An image of your muscles like a stretched, or twisted rubber band, relaxing and becoming limp may be helpful. Use any imagery that works for you. Relax the muscles all the way up your body from toes to head. You may fall asleep. It is likely that you will have a feeling of peaceful ease after this exercise. You can incorporate progressive body relaxation with all other techniques to create a more powerful starting point.

Notice as your daily life returns to your consciousness that the tensions return. Notice which life situation is associated with which tension.

Imagery

Imagery is important in all mind/body techniques. As a technical note, there is a difference between imagery and visualization: when you see a generic book in your mind's eye that is a visualization; when the book becomes a specific book that you have feelings about and that has a story attached, it is imagery.

As you approach any life challenge with the intent to heal it, it is helpful to first form a representation of the life challenge to interact with it. We have explored personifying life challenges, experiencing their energetic qualities, and discovering associated beliefs, emotional charges and physical attitudes. Each of these involves a different form of imagery. Each is a different abstract representation of the same life challenge. You can use any form of imagery to interact with and promote healing of any life challenge. For example, if in your mind's eye you see everything threatening as large and looming, you can make the situation less threatening by making the images small and distant, or fuzzy in black and white. If you have a fever, you might lower your body temperature by imagining yourself in a snow bank. Imagery is one way our minds express intent and receives guidance.

The automatic function of imagery theory states that by making an image, the unconscious mind begins to guide you toward the intended action or goal. You have deliver the intent in a form that your unconscious mind responds to. Your unconscious mind brings the necessary guidance and sensory feedback into your awareness to allow you to complete the intent.

A Safe Place

When using imagery, it is helpful to create a safe place or sanctuary. If you don't feel safe, you can't be aware of subtleties. When you don't feel safe, your body produces stress hormones in preparation for fight or flight and it's hard to go inside peacefully. Choose a place in your imagination where you are safe from outside influences. This may be in any form you wish. If you had a special safe place as a child, you can use this place. Some other possibilities are a garden, a safe house, a cloud or a cave.

The garden and the house are places that incorporate a representation of every aspect of a person - psychological, physical, intellectual and spiritual, and any other aspect of you that exists in any form. In these places you may make symbolical changes in your life. You may come here anytime. Make any imaginary changes you choose as often as necessary until they happen in your physical life. The choice of the place is a matter of what feels right to you at the time. You can change it at any time. Many people enjoy gardening. The images of planting, weeding and pruning are good images for expressing intent. Other people are not as comfortable in the outdoors. A house, cave or other protected place may feel safer. In these places you may summon the best authorities on any subject for opinions, directions or aid. You may call guides, allies, angels, dead relatives or any other resources you choose. You may create as many helpers as you choose to keep work going. You may use storehouses of spare body parts that can simply be snapped into place. You might find a control room that is the central place for directing changes in your body, mind and life. You may have, use or create anything you choose in your sanctuary to serve you in any way that you wish.

Another useful technique is to create an image of the future the way you would like it to be. Move forward in time one year and witness how your life is if you make no changes and just continue living and thinking in the same way. Move five years into the future, ten years, fifteen years and then twenty years. Witness these potential futures from a detached viewpoint, as if you were a neutral bystander. Now return to the present and create a different future. Experience a year from now as it would be if you did everything in your power to create the future that you want most. Step into the image and experience it as if it were real and happening right now. Take note of the action required to make it happen Move five years, ten years, fifteen years and twenty-five years into the future - experiencing it as it will be if you do everything you can to create the life you want.

You also may go to the past to make changes to affect the future. You might find it useful to return to a past trauma and change your belief about it and your relationship with it. For instance, if your father was an abusive alcoholic and constantly told you that you were worthless until you believed it, you may find it useful to return to the time when you accepted his judgment and change your mind. You can release this belief and the hold it has on your life now and in the future.

A useful guided meditation when working with a life challenge is, *Homecoming*, from John Bradshaw's book by the same name. In this meditative exercise you return to your childhood home, knock on the front door and collect your infant self, your toddler self, your preschool self, your grade school self, your adolescent self and your teenage self. You tell your parents that from now on you are going to take over parenting these parts of yourself because you are the only one who can really know their needs. Integrate each younger you into your body. Say goodbye to your parents and walk off into the sunset.

Another helpful guided meditation is from Virginia Satir called the, *Parts Party*. Imagine yourself sitting in a theater alone. Raise the curtain and begin to bring out parts of yourself represented as people. For example, you might represent the funny part as Josh Blue and the kind part as Mother Teresa. You might represent the tyrannical part as Attila the Hun. Bring out five parts of yourself that you like and have them stand on the right-hand side of the stage. Bring out five parts of yourself that you do not like and have them stand on the left-hand side of the stage. Go up onto the stage and look closely at each part from all angles and change them anyway you choose. After you have made the desired changes, have the parts merge with your body until each part has been changed and integrated. Please, no violence against your parts. They need your acceptance and respect. They have already been wounded. Why kick yourself when you're down?

When using imagery, the more clearly and accurately you can represent your life challenge, the more effective it will be. It is helpful to study everything you can about your life challenge, but it may be more powerful to study your own awareness of it. It is important to work with your medical support system to learn as much as possible about how your body works and how your life challenge exists with and inside your body. Medical people are the experts and can give you the clearest images of the dynamics of your body and your life challenge. They can help you to create a clear representation of your inner working with precision if you listen carefully and ask questions.

Remember that they are also human and could be wrong. You must use you own senses to find out if what they are telling you is accurate. If in doubt, get a second and third medical opinion. Check in with your own body as if you were an uninterested observer. We are masters at fooling ourselves about things we have emotions about. Be careful about mistaking judgments for observations. There are many anatomy and physiology apps that provide images and descriptions of the parts of your body and their functions.

When working with your life challenge, try seeing things from the larger view. It's easier to understand the ways your lifestyle contributes to maintaining or changing your life challenge if you consider how it relates to your family and friends. For example, it's easier to work with headaches if you know what triggers them. A headache may begin when your spouse, children or others begin talking about a certain subject. When you understand this dynamic cause and effect, you have the means to act to reduce your headaches. They become more than a tension and stabbing pain inside your head and you may now expand the experience of the tension and the pain to include the emotions, the beliefs and the previous trauma associated with the headaches. At some point, if you persist, it's likely you will find action that will change the situation so you no longer get headaches or they will become milder and less frequent.

You may also want to include other aspects related to your life challenge. Notice how your headaches exist in relation to yourself and others. Notice the tension in your muscles, nervous stomach, adrenaline rushes and other bodily signs of stress. The more you understand about your inner and outer worlds, the more likely you are to find the proper action leading to your ideal health, whatever that may be. Knowing how your headaches work may not result in a cure, but it may give you a little more control over what triggers and supports your headaches. If you understand that breathing a certain kind of dust in your workplace causes your headaches, you may choose to wear a dust mask. While you haven't cured the potential for headaches, you have removed or lessened an immediate cause of your headaches.

As your imagery of your life challenge grows clearer, you can actively and precisely direct your healing processes. We are such complex beings that we have no chance of ever discovering, let alone understanding, all the natural ways our bodies have of creating improved health. When using imagery, make up any way of working with your life challenge that you please and try it. It may not work, but chances are if you are able to find it in your imagination, it has a counterpart in reality and can be useful in your healing.

Make the most accurate representation you can of the inside of your body where the life challenge exists. Using your inner senses, see it, hear it, feel it, smell it and taste it. Know it as intimately as possible. Following the pain is a reliable way to follow a life challenge through your life as a whole, including the world outside. If you follow the pain, it will reveal to you things that contribute to it - situation, emotion, nutrition, abuses and so on. Change anything that your guidance suggests. Adjust your intent and imagery as you go. Constant adjustments may be necessary and only you can know what you're experiencing and what guidance is available to you.

Sometimes it is difficult to distinguish between innate guidance and wishful thinking. As you practice experiencing on a preverbal level, like a baby does before learning words and beliefs, you learn to be aware of increasingly subtle images and sensations. Innate guidance is a sensation and is as effortless as smelling. If you are struggling, or trying too hard, you are probably using wishful thinking instead of sensations based on true insight. With practice you can learn to recognize the difference. If you have doubts, it's probably wishful thinking.

A comparison test may help you. Think of a time when you found inner guidance. Represent this in any way you choose. You may see, feel, hear, smell or taste it. What works for you is what is important. Notice how this past experience fits into and feels inside your body. Compare that past experience and proven guidance with anything you have doubts about. Now, make up a similar guidance. Notice how the experience of the made-up guidance is different from the real thing and how these compare with the guidance in question.

Notice how this present doubtful guidance fits into and feels in your body. Check it against other times when you had inner guidance. Experience is the only way to learn this. New things are almost always difficult and practice always brings improvement. Be patient with yourself.

Using imagery, you may work indirectly with your life challenge. When you represent your life challenge as a child and interact with the child to help it get its emotional needs met, you are working indirectly with the physical manifestations of your life challenge. You are changing the emotional environment in which it exists. You may also work directly with the physical aspects.

Working directly with the messages of bodily sensations is simple and effective. Start by getting comfortable and bringing your awareness inward. Just notice, without judgment, what you find inside. Bring your awareness to the most present pain. If you find no pain, bring your awareness to an irritation (a small pain). If you find no irritation, bring your awareness to an itch or a tension (a smaller pain). Enter your body as if you were a tiny explorer able to maneuver anywhere. You will find any tools, supplies or helpers you may need as you move through your body.

Bring your awareness to the first area of concern and probe it. Feel it with tiny inner fingers and listen to it with an inner ear. See it, taste it, smell it and know it. Massage it with tiny fingers if that feels right. Call in helpers to remove wastes or make bodily repairs if needed. Stimulate the area with sound, light or heat. Soothe with color, tone, coolness or imagery. Use any pleasant sensory image you want. Add a theme song to keep the work happy. Supervise repair or remodeling. Use your imagination in any way that feels right. This is what imagery is, using your imagination.

Light

Working in the body with images of light is a powerful technique. Russian scientists have studied biophotons or light that each cell of a human body is believed to emit. Biophotons can be tuned to any measurable light frequency, thus, each cell of your body can use any color of light as a defense. An ultraviolet light can be emitted to kill bacteria, a harsh red orange color or infrared to kill viruses or a honey-colored light to kill some anaerobic intestinal parasites. Biophotons can be emitted as a soft glow, a laser sharp beam or anything in between.

A hot, white light might be imagined as cauterizing the blood supply to a tumor to starve it. This image may be used for repairing a tear or cut, or cleaning a clogged artery. The image may be experienced as bright static electricity - like intense and focused sparks, a constant laser like beam or a pulsed light. Always use what feels right to you.

Light may be imagined as a constant glow that surrounds an area or organ. For example, if you are HIV-positive, you might experience the bone marrow bathed deeply in a harsh red orange light that penetrates and kills the virus in the white blood cells. White light is effective for pain control and for containing the spread of toxic organisms or substances. Always tune the color and its characteristics to make it right for your present use. The right color may change from minute-to-minute or day-to-day.

When using light in any form, always release excess light from your body when you are finished. Your body will tell you how much of the light is excess. Trust it. White light, like any agent that relieves pain, also can mask it and hide the sensory feedback that may guide you to permanent relief of the pain. Re-injury may occur as a result of hiding the pain and its guidance.

The safest way to use light imagery in healing is always to start with an image of weak, crystal clear light. Using clear light involves no danger of masking or overloading. The image of adding a more intense clear light glow to your body, or in your body, allows for healing intent to begin working. While probing with and directing clear light, it's possible that you will feel the innate guidance to add the use of color. Let that guidance choose the color to use. When using color, always tune it to the exact right qualities for your use. This may require constant adjustment. Follow your innate guidance to find the exact right color and method of delivering it. Trust yourself. This is the most direct and effective use of light imagery.

One method of choosing the color of light for a given situation is to bring your awareness to the area you are working with. When you have a clear awareness of your current life challenge and you hold a clear intent in your mind to heal it, with your eyes closed place a finger on your forehead and notice what color you see. If you are working with a headache, you may see red. You may have a feeling that this red would be best delivered by pumping it through your blood. The next time you have a headache, even though it might feel the same, you might see yellow and have the urge to breathe it into your brain.

Color has proven to be effective in treating intestinal parasites and yeast infections. You may find guidance to soak your entire body in golden light one day. The next day you may feel that attacking the individual parasites with purple laser beams is the best method. Trust yourself. If you think you may be following wishful thinking, use a comparison test. Experiment with color and fine tune it as you work.

Use colored light with movement, breath or sound. Each sense or capacity you focus with increases the effectiveness of your conscious involvement in your healing. The following exercises combines breath and movement with light and imagery. The most effective use of any of these tools is what feels right to you.

Bone Marrow Cleansing

Stand comfortably with knees slightly bent and feet at shoulder wide. Take a moment to quiet your body. As you inhale, allow your arms to float effortlessly upwards at your sides like wings until they reach shoulder height with palms facing outward. For just a moment, imagine your feet reaching to the center of the earth and your head reaching to the stars. Imagine your arms reaching out into the universe. Exhale and let your arms gently float down until they meet in front of your abdomen forming an upright bowl. Let your hands rise to your navel holding the bowl as you inhale. Turn your hands outward as they pass your navel and let them continue to rise until they form a bowl over your head with the palms pointing up. Breathe intense white light into the bowl until it is overflowing.

Turn your palms toward the top of your head while you exhale. Imagine pouring the white light from the bowl through the top of your head. Push the light slowly through the center of your bones. As the light moves down through your body, imagine pushing dark wastes deep into the earth. Repeat three times and release the excess light.

A variation is to continue to expand the white light using the breath to intensify the light. With each breath, imagine your skeleton glowing brighter until the light begins to push dark wastes through the pores of your skin. Continue to push the wastes out until white light shines from every pore. Release the excess light.

Organ Cleansing and Charging

In the practice of Qigong, there are five reservoir organs of energy. They are called the five jewels: kidneys, liver, spleen, lungs and heart. These organs may be cleaned, charged and rejuvenated with colored light.

Get in a comfortable position with your back straight. Bring your awareness to the organ with which you are working. Start with your kidneys. The exercise is the same for each organ, only the colors differ. Imagine with each inhaling breath through your nose you bring a sapphire blue, or deep blue black, color into your kidneys and swish it around. With each exhaling breath release the air, darkened with the wastes from the kidneys, through your mouth. Continue bringing in the blue and releasing the wastes using slow deep abdominal breaths until you release all the wastes and the color is pure and bright.

Continue cleansing and charging each organ using pearl white for the lungs, topaz yellow for your spleen, emerald green for your liver, ruby red for your heart and sapphire blue for your kidneys.

Core of Energy

Get comfortable with your back straight. Bring your awareness to your breathing and begin to breathe deeply into your pelvic floor. Imagine a central core of intense energy spinning as it rises through your pelvic floor up through the crown of your head. Feel this column of energy spinning faster and growing more intense with each breath. Begin to draw all wastes from your body and mind into the core where they burn and are released as mist from the rising column. Continue until you find no more waste material to release. These wastes may be physical, emotional, energetic, spiritual or any other kind.

Make it Fun

Imagery can be effective in any form you choose. Use imagery that is uniquely your own if it occurs to you. Make it fun in any way that suits you. The little boy who started it all in the Boston hospital played a fun game to heal his tumor. Anything that makes your imagery more engaging for you is helpful. It's your body. You're the one in it. Choose to make your experience of it rich.

Participating in Your Medical Treatment

Unlimited ways exist for using mind/body techniques to intensify other healing treatments. Here are a few specific techniques for helping with, participating in or guiding medical treatments. The techniques that are easiest for you will be the most effective.

The most common treatment a physician uses is medication in the form of a pill, liquid, salve or injection. Ask lots of questions about the medication. What does it do and how does it do it? What side effects may occur? What are the desired effects and why are they desirable? The more information you have the better. If a pill is relieving a headache by causing blood vessels in your head to relax and expand allowing increased blood flow, it is helpful to follow the process from beginning to end. You might see and feel the pill as you swallow it. Notice the feelings in your body and your emotions as you put it in your mouth. Has anything changed by your choice to take the pill or in the act of swallowing it?

How you feel about the drug influences how well it works. Studies show things like the color of the pill, or the presence of a smiley face on a Band-Aid, or how you feel about your medical team, can accelerate or hinder healing. Choosing an attitude of taking control and making the drug do what it is intended to do while protecting your body from side effects will increase the efficacy of the treatment. You can also learn to cause the desired effect of the treatment using your natural resources in many cases. If you have excess stomach acid you can learn to have your body produce the appropriate amount of acid rather than taking a chemical to neutralize the acid.

Follow the pill as it dissolves and migrates into your bloodstream. If one possible side effect of the medication is stomach irritation, protect your stomach with something like a buttery coating, or use a vibration or sound to prevent the drug from touching the lining of your stomach. Follow the medication as it moves in just seconds through your blood into your brain. Notice how you react to the pill as it breaks up and moves through your body. In any instance where you find an undesirable side effect, even if it isn't a listed side effect, do something to protect yourself. Protect your body in whatever way you can. Boost the effectiveness of the medication with other aids at your disposal such as relaxing, increasing natural body chemicals, using light, sound, breath, imagery or anything else that occurs to you.

As you receive injections, you might relax and follow the needle experiencing it easily and painlessly penetrating your skin and muscle. Experience a hole opening to receive it. Then follow the liquid through your body, noticing reactions and directing resources to reduce side effects and increase the treatments success. Channel the drug directly to the place where it's needed.

If the intent of the medication is to kill an invading force, such as bacteria, imagine it destroying the bacteria. You may choose to kill the bacteria with sound and light along with the drug. You may choose to change the chemical balances so that the bacteria cannot survive or direct the white blood cells in an assault on the invaders. You may choose to protect the beneficial bacteria from the antibiotic. It is against some people's beliefs to use such violent images. If this is the case, you might use images of gathering up the bacteria and removing it unharmed. Work within your reality. The scope of your reality will change as you choose to claim more self-awareness, self-respect and self-determination. This is a natural evolution of consciousness.

If the intent of the medication is to change chemical or

electrical imbalances, experience these changes happening as the drug reaches the target area of your body. Choose for the imbalances to change in the exact right way.

If the intent of the medication is to kill cells in the body, as with chemotherapy or radiation therapy, guide the drug or radiation to the targeted, diseased cells. Shield the healthy cells, not allowing the chemical or radiation to touch them. You may choose to use images of pipelines, tanker trucks or aircraft to deliver the agent precisely to the offending cells. You may choose images of light pathways and sound barriers. Use any imagery that appeals to you.

You may use these techniques for participating in surgery or other medical procedures. You may choose to remain aware during surgery on some level and monitor the operation for signs of complications. Even under total anesthesia, some people are aware of events in the operating room. You may use imagery to rehearse the operation including your choice to control blood flow, heart rate, respiration, blood pressure, or other aspects of your physiology.

While rehearsing, you might find it helpful to set the scene of the operation in your sanctuary rather than the hospital. This gives you an increased feeling of control. If your surgeon is cooperative, you may want to have her talk to you during the procedure and keep you informed about what your body needs to do to help at all times. It's also helpful to rehearse the operation with your surgeon or surgical nurse.

Imagine feeling and helping with each step. Follow each procedure in your mind and body. Imagine stopping the flow of blood to the area of the operation. Prelive the entire operation, from leaving home and entering the hospital to the time of complete healing. This process helps to reduce fear and trauma associated with the surgery or treatment.

When working with an acupuncturist, body worker, chiropractor, physical therapist, physician, psychiatrist, psychotherapist or any other health care professional, have them tell you what they are doing and what outcome they are trying to achieve. Have them explain how and why it is desirable to do what they are doing. You can make this work faster, easier and more effective if you actively participate. What you can do by choice may amaze you.

You can adapt these techniques to any life challenge. You are the source of your best guidance. When you take charge of your healing process you increase your chances for the best outcome. Treat yourself gently and respectfully. Within your own body and your own experience you can find amazing abilities and insight. Take control. It's your body and you're the one in it.

ABOUT THE AUTHOR

A motorcycle accident that threatened to leave Carl Brahe paralyzed led him on a healing journey that saved him from life in a wheelchair and continues more than 30 years later making him stronger and healthier in every aspect of his life. Part of the process was earning a master's degree in psychology, actually a master's degree in his personal healing. In his writings he shares the tools gained from study with many exceptional holistic and native healers, energy workers and medical professionals from western and traditional Chinese medicine and mind/body therapists. Carl currently resides in the mountains outside of Denver, CO.

www.ingramcontent.com/pod-product-compliance
Lightning Source LLC
Chambersburg PA
CBHW021210290526
45796CB00005B/25